YAK HUSBANDRY

YAK HUSBANDRY

By

GOUTAM MONDAL
BISWAJIT ROY
&
BISWAJIT BRAHMA

SSPH

SATISH SERIAL PUBLISHING HOUSE
403, Express Tower, Commercial Complex, Azadpur, Delhi-110033 (India)
Phone : 011-27672852, Fax : 91-11-27672046
E-mail :info@satishserial.com, hkjain1975@yahoo.com
Website : www.satishserial.com

Published by :

SATISH SERIAL PUBLISHING HOUSE
403, Express Tower, Commercial Complex, Azadpur, Delhi-110033 (INDIA)
Phone : 011-27672852 Fax : 91-11-27672046
E-mail : info@satishserial.com, hkjain1975@yahoo.com

Print Again : 2023

ISBN : 978-93-81226-27-8

Composed, Designed & Printed in India

PREFACE

Yak (*Poephagus grunniens*) is a sturdy animal of higher elevations. Yak are predominantly find in Tibet, Mongolia, part of India, Bhutan, Pakistan, Russia etc. They are acclimatized to harsh and often unfriendly climatic conditions with minimum availability of feed materials for their survival. They have the specific adaptive characters to adapt those situations like coat colour, fibre production, compact and sturdy body shape, larger thoracic cavity and lungs, browsing and grazing habit, sure footed and pack performance in steep mountains, which is not present in other species and make them most suitable to live in high altitudes. Yak population in India is 83,000 though it signifies a religious and cultural sentiment of millions of people around the world (population is more than 10 millions worldwide). It implies the prosperity of people in Tibetan Buddhism and some part of India. Yak is a multi-purpose animal, which play important role in the human civilization at a very high altitude. Due to some reasons like hybridization with local hilly cows, poaching, mechanization in transport and agriculture, population of yak declining very fast in some parts of India. So, there is an urgent need to conserve the species.

In this book 'Yak Husbandry', nutrition, management and reproduction have been discussed in detail. At the same time, origin and distribution, adaptation, behaviour is discussed with special reference to yak. Performance of pure yak and hybrids (crosses of yak and cow) and diseases usually encountered by the farmers have also been discussed in this book. The information of this book could be of use for the students, researcher any person willing to know about the wonder animal. Such information at a simplest form is presented in the book and hardly to be found in such a concise form for the wide range of readers, academicians and researchers.

Goutam Mondal
Biswajit Roy
Biswajit Brahma

CONTENTS

Preface v

Chapter 1 : Introduction 1
- Yak: A wonder animal, 1
- Yak has many names, 2
- Yak in human civilization, 3

Chapter 2 : Origin and Distribution 7
- Systematics and phylogeny, 7
- The *bovini* tribe: yak and its relative, 8
- Origin and domestication , 11
- Breeds of yak, 12
- Distribution, 18

Chapter 3 : Adaptation to Cold Climate 21
- Introduction, 21
- Adaptive mechanisms, 24
  - Anatomical/ structural adaptations, 24
  - Physiological adaptation, 29
  - Behavioural adaptation, 33
  - Reproductive adaptation, 36
  - Metabolic adaptation, 38

Chapter 4 : Reproduction 39
- Reproductive organs, 41
  - Female reproductive organs, 41
  - Male reproductive organs, 46
- Reproductive endocrinology, 50
  - Endocrine glands, 50
  - Reproductive hormones, 53

Reproductive processes, 65
Puberty, 65
Sperm and Semen, 68
Follicular development, 73
Female reproductive cycle, 77
Gestation, 83
Assisted reproductive technologies (ART) in yak, 87

Chapter 5 : Nutrition 97
Classification of feeds, 98
Roughage, 98
Concentrate, 100
Unconventional feeds, 103
Functions of nutrients, 103
Water, 103
Carbohydrate, 105
Protein, 114
Lipids, 123
Minerals, 131
Vitamins, 134
Nutrient requirement of yak for various stages of life, 136
Energy requirement for maintenance, growth and lactation, 136
Protein requirement for maintenance, growth and lactation, 137
Forage availability and pasture management, 137

Chapter 6 : Management of Yak 143
Yak: body conformation, 145
Acclimatization in high altitudes, 146
Management of animal, 147
Calf rearing, 147
Rearing of heifers, 152
Rearing of pregnant animals, 153
Rearing of lacting animals, 154
Management of male yak, 160
Routine farm management, 161
Herd management, 162
Controlling the herd, 163
Tethering, 163
Housing, 164
Restraining, 166
Culling of yak, 166

Feeding salt, 167
Barter system of marketing of product of yak, 167
Yak management activity schedule, 167
Dentition and determination of age, 170

Chapter 7 : Production Performance 175
Growth, 175
Factors affecting growth, 179
Meat production, 181
Meat quantity, 181
Effect of age and sex, 182
Meat quality, 183
Draught performance, 186
Milk production, 187
Milk from different species, 189
Milk biosynthesis, 190
Precursors of milk, 191
Factors affecting milk composition, 192
Milk production in a second year without calving again, 196
Factors influencing milk yield, 197
Fibre production, 199
Fibres and staple properties, 200
Hides, 202
Conservation of pure yak, 202

Chapter 8 : Hybridization and Performance of Hybrids 209
Introduction, 209
Purpose of hybridization, 210
Nomenclature of the various progenies, 212
Production performance of hybrids, 212
Growth, 212
Meat production, 214
Milk production, 215
Draught and work performance, 217
Reproduction and fertility, 218
Female reproduction, 218
Male reproduction, 220

Chapter 9 : Behaviour 223
Association and social behaviour, 224
Reactive behaviour, 225

Sexual behaviour, 226
Male, 226
Female, 227
Parturient behaviour, 228
Neonatal behaviour, 229
Ingestive behaviour, 230
Ingestive / exploratory behaviour, 232
Epimelatic (car giving) behaviour, 233
Resting behaviour, 233

Chapter 10 : Diseases of Yak 235
Viral diseases, 236
Infectious Bovine Rhinotracheitis (IBR), 237
Rinderpest, 237
Viral diarrhoea/mucosal disease, 238
Bacterial diseases, 238
Anthrax, 238
Brucellosis, 239
Colibacillosis, 240
Leptospirosis, 240
Mastitis, 241
Haemorrhagic septisemia, 241
Salmonellosis, 242
Tuberculosis, 242
Contagious bovine pleuropneumonia, 242
Parasitic diseases, 242
Endoparasites, 243
Metabolic and deficiency diseases, 244
Bloat, 244
Acidosis, 245
Ketosis, 245
Milk fever, 246
Grass tetany, 247
Mineral and trace element deficiency, 247

Chapter 11 : Future Research and Conclusion 251

Chapter 1

Introduction

1.1 Yak: A wonder animal

Yak *(Poephagus grunniens)*, a close relative of cattle, is one of the world's most remarkable domestic ruminant as it thrives in conditions of extreme harshness and unfriendly weather conditions while providing a livelihood security for people of high altitudes. Long wooly hair makes them very attractive and it is necessary for thriving in their natural habitat at altitudes of 3000-5000 m or more as in Tibetan plateau and part of Arunachal Pradesh, Sikkim and Ladakh region of Jammu & Kashmir, Lahul and Spiti of Himachal Pradesh. The distinctive grunt produced by these animals during mating season gives them the systematic name of *Poephagus grunniens.* Yak is a very sturdy animal and may negotiate and graze in areas normally inaccessible to hardiest cattle breed.

A range of physiological adaptations viz. thick hide, subcutaneous fat layer, dense hair, large heart, lungs and a high erythrocyte count make these animals to survive under extreme cold and to tolerate the low oxygen content in the air of high altitude. As their habitat is sloppy mountain terrain, they survive without any slip or injury due to their surefootedness characteristics. Probably they are most surefooted mountain domesticated animal. They can proceed without stumbling along the worst mountain paths, with a wall of rock on one side and a void on the other but without ever falling. Yak's sense of smell is excellent, although its eye sight is only mediocre. Since their domestication, probably by ancient Qiang people of China, yak played a multidimensional role in social and cultural life of central Asian mountainous civilization. An important pack animal of high altitude, yak also produces valuable animal products like milk, meat, hide, fibre, dung and many local products. Yaks are presently distributed in high altitude of China, Mongolia, Kazakhstan, Tuva, Russia, India, Pakistan and Bhutan. In India, yaks are found in the states of Arunachal Pradesh, Sikkim, Jammu & Kashmir, nothern part of Uttar Pradesh, Uttaranchal and Himachal Pradesh and contribute an important role in socio-economic as well as religious life of people in the region. Interspecies mating of yak and cow is possible (2n= 60 for both the species) and are extensively practiced in lower mountainous ranges of these regions. Most of the drought operations are carried out by these animals, since mechanization in agriculture has not been possible due to steep and rouged terrain of these regions. The common saying '*what moves Tibet and Mongolia does do on yaks*' indicate the importance of yak in high altitude regions. It is well adapted to the place where literally there is no or little vegetation for survivability of animals. However, despite their diverse role in human civilization, the recent trend has indicated that their population is decreasing at an alarming rate, which has been a serious concern for both yak farmers and conservation scientists. The major difficulty with research on yak remains the inaccessibility or limited accessibility to their natural habitat which is extremely harsh. Nevertheless, recently, research on yak including modern biotechniques for conservation and improvement of production efficiency, has taken pace and this wonder animal has shown considerable scope of improvement through these biotechniques.

1.2 Yak has many names

The term "yak" has probable origin from "yag"- a Tibetan equivalent for yak bull with *dri* the equivalent Tibetan term for the female yak. In Ladakh region of India, yak is called as 'yag'. Other languages follow this name closely. The ancient Chinese people called the animal *Ya Niu*, denoting the yak's large body, outstretched horns, long hair and big tail. In time, the name was reduced to a word pronounced as 'ya'. Local name of wild yak is *Tibetan dong* or *brong dong*. In Hindi, wild and domesticated yak are called as *chour gau* and *ban chour*, respectively. Interspecies hybrids of yak and cattle are generally called as *zo* and *zomo, gar* and *garmo, de* and *demo, tor* and *tormo* etc. to the F_1, F_2 F_3 and F_4 generation male and female, respectively, although these names vary from region to region. The hybrid males are invariably sterile, while the females are fertile.

1.3 Yak in human civilization

Yak farming is closely associated with the social and cultural life of the people, most particularly in the vast rangeland grazing areas of the Tibetan Plateau and other parts around the Himalayan mountain range of higher altitudes. The yak is, moreover, a component of the religious practices and manifestations of Tibetan Buddhism. Yak production has an impact in the economy of Ladakh region. To meet the challenges of a harsh and often unfriendly environment in the region, farmers have developed a system of using common grazing lands, mostly in the high hills during summer with other ruminants, for the most part in a nomadic fashion resulting in rotational use of the grazing lands. Much of this developed through agreements between families in a particular village. However, these are stall fed during the harsh winter months when the place is covered with thick snow and supplemented with lucerne hay, barley and wheat straw with occasional feeding of barley, wheat, buck wheat grain and detoxified apricot oilcake to pregnant and lactating female yak. With the more recent moves towards a market-oriented economy, changes have been observed with the rearing of yak as most of the drought work was effectively and efficiently done by mechanical power and thus people changing their mindset to cross the animals with cow for better milk production, resulting decreasing in number of yak population throughout the region, even in India.

Yak is an useful animal in the high altitudes as these can carry heavier loads than other animals (around 150 kg), give meat in the lean period, milk with high fat content (10.9 percent) and hide and hair for winter clothing (500 g down hair and 1200 g coarse hair annually), preparation of tents, horns for manufacturing milking pails and various decorating materials. Rearing of these animals requires less attention as well as they can well survive and produce well under harsh climatic condition of high altitudes. There was a great demand of bushy tail in the past. Stalked on wooden handle mounted with carved silver cover the chawar of yak tail is used in temples of royal families. These are also used in important ceremonies in many yak rearing countries viz., India, Bhutan, Nepal, Tibet, Turkey, Mongolia and China. One of the most important purpose of rearing yak is to produce hybrids crossing with cattle and mithun for obtaining higher milk, fat, flesh and better draught animals.

Yak population in India are scattered and there is urgent need to type characterization of the species inhabiting different places and to ascertain the genetic diversity among them. Type characterization should include important confrontation traits, traits of production and reproduction and also biochemical and physiological parameters. Genetic diversity can be studied by both univariate and multivariate analysis approach. Study of genetic diversity among these population vis-a- vis other species of bovidae family using protein and DNA markers also be needed under our condition. At a time when the country is fast moving forward on all fronts influenced by a market driven economy, there has been tremendous widening of earning avenues to the people even in far-flung inaccessible areas – the habitat of yak. Yak products like milk by products, meat by products, horn and hooves, skin and hide and most importantly hair must be commercialized in the region. Yak are facing danger as often the younger population is showing interest for other avenues like small business or tourist guide that are readily available and giving money in a shorter period of time. This indicates the rearing of yak must be make more profitable and market oriented by the scientists working in the field. At the same time shrinkage of habitat due to deforestation, industrialization, increased human population may be other attributes for decline yak population in India. The traditional open seasonal migratory system of yak rearing is today confined to particular areas due to restrictions placed on movement by the different tribal community and also due to the restrictions on trans-boundary movement. A considerable part of the high hills in the yak rearing places is stony and difficult for grazing with only few pockets of small meadow and availability of water. Habitat restoration and its improvement for supporting yak as a whole should get attention by the government. Grazing land in the mid altitude hills as well as high altitude should be improved by fertilization or by other means so that availability of fodder for yak is increased.

Role of yak in the high altitudes as earlier said as a pack animal and its adaptability in the cold weather is unparallel. Its worth as a producer of milk (mostly as a crossbred), meat, hide, hair/ wool and dung as fuel in extreme living conditions is also commendable. The research is thus needed to conserve the yak and improvement of economic trait of the animal and survival of the species and livelihood security of people related to it. Genetic improvement may be done through selection of superior bull by progeny testing. Though under nomadic system of yak rearing it is very difficult, elite animals may be done by individual performance, pedigree and type conformity. Once elite herd of yak is established, then it is very easy to genetic improvement of yak. At the same time, interspecies hybridization may be done to improve the milk production. This is important for farmers' economic point of view. However, male hybrids are always sterile with higher draught power and females are higher milk producer and this is one of the most important factor for declining pure yak population in India.

Yak milk has known to have therapeutic and medicinal value due to physiologically active component as maintained on grasses, natural fodders and other fauna under organic system by default mostly in higher elevations. Therapeutic and medicinal quality of milk, meat and other byproducts needs to be investigated scientifically and at the same time traditional old age practice of processing the products into byproducts needs to be investigated for improvement. Though most of the farmers are growing the yak or other livestock in the high altitudes of India 'organic' one, extension activities are needed to aware the people about importance of organic and sustainable livestock farming for the improvement of the economic condition. Technologies developed for the rural masses by National Research Centre on Yak, India viz., small yak milk processing unit for demonstration, system analysis and training to rural youth, technologies for production of value added milk products from yak like dahi, paneer, khoa, flavoured milk and lassi, whey beverages and milk sweets which can increase the income by many folds. The technologies need to be propagated in yak rearing places for entrepreneurship among the rural youth and small farmers.

To improve the milk production from yak crosses, pure yak population is declining in many states and genetic improvement for conserving the yak is needed keeping in mind its uniqueness in survivability in higher elevations, multiple use for milk, meat, hide, fibre and above all inevitability of yak to the high altitude people under prevailing cultural, religious and socio-economic conditions. Yak is living in a very harsh and often unfriendly, fragile eco-system, the natural selection has played a pivotal role in yak breeding. There is wide variability in various traits in yak, which has to be properly utilized for their improvement. Milk yield (daily to total lactation yield), lactation length, milk composition, growth for maximum meat production (from birth weight to dressing percentage, lean meat yield, feed conversion for growth), fibre production (hair yield, down fibre yield and fineness), drought power and reproductive performance are the economically important traits and have to be substantially improved without affecting the adaptability by using suitable breeding strategies for improving the economic status of the farmers. Outside the conservation zone, the hybridization of yak with low producing hill cattle or zebu cattle is widely practiced among the farmers so as to harvest maximum milk from both the ancestors and sterile male for drought/ work purpose. This hybridization has some advantages which is milk and drought purpose but at the same time reduces the adaptability of the offspring and survivability is poor as compared to pure yak in higher altitudes.

Management of domestic yak is migratory one during the summer months when yak are grazed on high hills along with sheep, goat, ponies etc., whereas during winter months stall feeding is practiced. During stall feeding period, lucerne hay, wheat and barley straw and *chapatti* or other kitchen waste to the pregnant and early lactating animals is given. This is to provide more milk to the farmer from the yak, and to support value addition domestically.

Yak is multipurpose animal and living in harsh and often unfriendly environment provides livelihood security to the millions of people in trans-himalayan range and research is needed to improve the economic condition of the people as well as genetic improvement, hybridization, growth, milk and meat production with low inputs. Conservation is also needed keeping the view in mind the sharp decline of the yak population globally.

□□□

Chapter 2

Origin and Distribution

Yak along with cattle, buffalo, sheep and goat, constitute one of the most important group of ruminants that has been domesticated. Their specialized digestive system enables them to utilize cellulose from roughages as an energy source to produce valuable animal products. In addition, since the period from Neolithic transition, period when the majority of humanity changed from a huntergatherer existence to a sedentary agricultural lifestyle, these animals have become an integral part of livelihood and food security of people. Even today in the age of mechanized agriculture, animals like yak and its hybrids are mainstay for agricultural operations and carriage in hilly terrains of some parts of China, India, Pakistan and many other developing countries. This chapter describes the zoological classification of yaks and their close relatives, their origin and domestication process as well as their range of distribution in the present world.

2.1 Systematics and Phylogeny

Yak belongs to the *Bovidae* family within the order *Artiodactyala* or even-toed ungulates which also includes larger group such as the antelopes, cattle, sheep and goats. The oldest fossils of Artiodactyls have been found to be 50-60 million years old. A subgroup within this order is *Ruminantia*, a group characterized by its specialized digestive system with multi-compartmental stomach and ability to utilize grass and leaves as energy source. The *Bovidae* family of *Artiodactyala* order (subgroup: *Ruminantia*) first appeared around 20 million years ago and underwent a rapid radiation which is considered to have been unparalleled in other large mammals (Gatesy *et al.*, 1997). The bovidae group comprises around 100 animal species and is characterized by presence of permanent hollow horns. The *bovidae* family, based on archaeological and molecular studies, has been divided into five to nine subfamilies. There is no general agreement on exact number of subfamilies, but acknowledged subfamilies include Bovinae (cattle, buffalo, yak, nilgai etc.), Cephalophinae (duikers), Caprinae (sheep and goats), Hippotraginae (roan antilope) and Antilopinae (gazelles) (Lenstra and Bradley, 1999). The Bovinae subfamily has been divided in several tribes, the largest being the Bovini tribe. This tribe started to diverge around 4 million years ago and encompasses wild and domesticated cattle, buffalo, yak and bison. Although, genera classification within bovini tribe has also been a subject of controversy, it is obvious that three diverse group i.e. *Bos* (cattle, yak, gaur, bantang, kouprey), Buffalo (bubalina and syncerina) and bison (bison, wisent) constitute this tribe (Figure 2.1). Yak has been classified under genus *Bos* or sometime it has been placed under a separate genus *Poephagus*. All the members of *Bos* and Bison group has similar chromosome number (2n=60), except gaur (2n=58). The buffalo group has different chromosome number (2n= 52, 50, 48 for African, water and Swamp buffalo, respectively) and thus interspecies mating has been restricted to *Bos* and Bison groups. Interspecies hybridization of cattle x yak produces viable offspring. The male hybrids of this cross, however, are sterile.

The present day molecular data, however, suggest a much diverse classification within the bovini tribe. This has led to the hypothesis that geographical factors along with pattern of spread of ancestral civilization have determined the extent of genetic exchange among the ancient animal population which is articulated through genetic similarity amongst these animals.

2.2 The *bovini* tribe: Yaks and its relative

The mammalian tribe bovini (subfamily: bovinae, family: bovidae) comprises world's most important domesticated group of animals

(Figure 2.1). Domesticated cattle, the most popular species of *Bovini* tribe, have now two recognized forms; the humpless *taurine* cattle of Europe, West Africa and northern Asia, (*Bos taurus*) and the humped *zebu* cattle of southern Asia and Africa (*Bos indicus*). The word "zebu" has probably originated from Tibetan *zea* or *zeba,* meaning camel hump or from *gebo* or *geba,* the Portuguese for humped. Distribution of these animals over different climatic zone has resulted in distinct morphological and physiological differences. *Bos indicus* cattle, which inhabit the hot arid or semi-arid regions of Asia and Africa, have lower basal metabolic rate, more active sweat glands and are more resistant to ticks and intestinal parasites than taurine cattle. Zebu cattle have a different vocal sound from taurine cattle and also possess a much stronger herd instinct. Their most well-known morphological

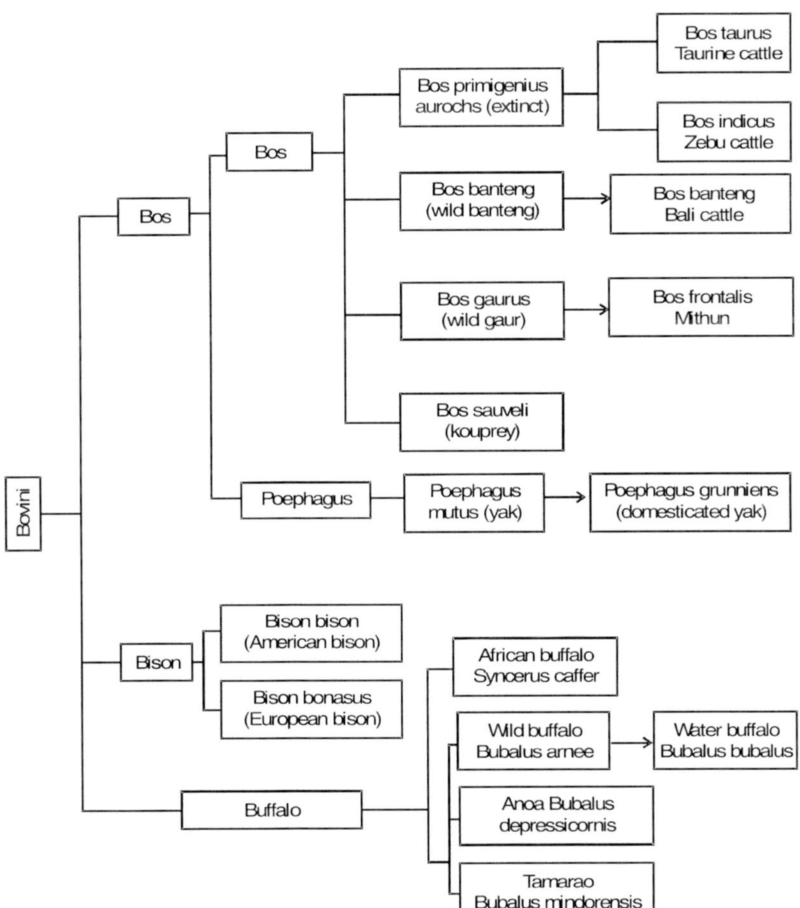

Figure 2.1 : The Bovini tribe and its descendants

differences with taurine cattle are presence of a hump either in a thoracic or cervico-thoracic position, a pendulous dewlap and a navel flap. *Bos taurus* cattle on the other hand, are usually confined to temperate zones with higher levels of rainfall and denser vegetation. Some of the taurine breeds of cattle are famous milk producer of the world (e.g. Holstein, Brown Swiss, Ayreshire etc.).

Two genera in the bovini tribe, Syncerina (African buffalo) and Bubalina (*Bubalus* species, water buffalo, arni, tamarao and anoa) constitute the buffalo group. It is believed that buffaloes were first tamed and then domesticated for agricultural operations in 5000 B.C. in China, in 2500 B.C. in Mesopotamia during the period of Akkadian dynasty and in Indus valley civilization of Indian subcontinent extending to Harappa, Mohanjodaro and some parts of Gujarat, Rajasthan and Haryana. While some species are domesticated (*Bubalus bubalus, Bubalus carabanesis* etc.) others are still wild (*Syncerus caffer, Bubalus arnee*) and difficult to be tamed. Two types of water buffalo have been discerned that differ in karyotypes: the swamp type of South East Asia and river type of Indian subcontinent. The anoa (*Bubalus [Anoa] depressicornis*) is the smallest bovine species that lives in the forests of Indonesia. Tamarao (*Bubalus [Anoa] mindorensis*) is also smaller than water buffalo that inhabit in the southern Philippine island. Most of the world buffalo (water buffalo) are found in Asia with some well defined breeds of India, Pakistan (riverine type) and China (swamp type). A significant proportion is also found in Egypt, Italy and Brazil.

The bison, sometime taken for buffalo as a misnomer, are the wild cattle of North American Prairie region. The American (*Bison bison*) and European (*B. bonasus*) bison are the largest terrestrial mammals in North America and Europe. Bison are herd animals and are nomadic grazers. Both species were hunted close to extinction during the 19th and 20th centuries but have since rebounded, although the European bison is still endangered. Inter-species hybridization is possible with cattle and the hybrid has been called as beefalo.

The yaks (*Poephagus [Bos] grunniens*) are long-haired bovine found throughout the Himalayan region of south Central Asia, the Qinghai-Tibetan Plateau and as far north as Mongolia. Their typical grunting during mating season has given them the systematic name *Bos grunniens.* In addition to a large domestic population, there is a small, vulnerable wild yak population. In fact wild yak's existence is one of continuous struggle against the adverse forces of its environment. It is one of the highest dwelling animals in the world. In summer time yaks are found at elevations ranging from 4000 to 6000 metres and even in winter they do not descend much below this level. The colour of wild yak is a uniform blackish brown with a little white about the muzzle. On the other hand, the domestic yaks usually have patches of white on the chest and tail. This tendency to piebald (combination of two colours especially with white and black patches) is never seen in the wild species. Domestic yaks are at times wholly black and like wild yaks, wander to great heights in search of food.

Three wild species banteng (*Bos banteng*), gaur or Indian bison (*Bos gaurus*), gayal (*Bos frontalis*) and their descendents form a group in bovini tribe. While small population of wild banteng inhabit in South East Asia and Java. Bali cattle, a descendent of wild banteng have a fair population in the islands of Bali and other parts of Indonesia. Bali cattle are reputed for their heat tolerant capacity and exceptional quality of meat. Gaurs are found in the eastern states of India, Indonesia and China. Domestication of gayal took place around 500 B.C. and the domesticated animals are known as mithun. These animals are human friendly and are found in eastern states of India. Inter-species cross of gayal and gaur with cattle has been reported in some literature where, heterosis has been observed in F1 hybrids.

2.3 Origin and domestication

Although plenty of research, including both archaeological and molecular genetics studies have been done to find out origin of domesticated cattle and buffalo, information on origin of domesticated yak are sparse. Existence of a yak pastoral system in Qinghai Tibetan Plateau is well established dating back to 4500 years BC, but most researchers believe that domestication event took place around 10000 years BC. Domestic yak were derived from wild yak for production of wool, milk, meat and for normal work. Archeological data evidences that domestication of yak has been done around 5000 year ago by ancient Qiang people in north Tibet (Wiener *et al.*, 2003). Since, it is difficult to distinguish between wild and domesticated yak fossils, this however, can not be affirmed without definite evidence. The earliest *Poephagus* fossils found so far, dates back to lower Pleistocene age (Flerow, 1980). Several studies indicates that this was the time when genetic divergence took place between *Poephagus* and its sister group *Bison bison,* some 1.8 millions years ago. Molecular evidences suggest at least two main lineages in domestic yak diverged around 1.0 million years ago (Guo *et al.*, 2006), much earlier before yak was domesticated. This tempts the assumption that two independent origin of domestication might have taken place for yak. However, there are strong molecular evidences that all domesticated yaks results from a single wild population (Guo *et al.*, 2006). It has been suggested that around 86000 to 157000 years BC, several cycles of glacial and interglacial climatic oscillation drove the yak into two refugia, where population divergence occurred. They meet again during interglacial or post glacial period and population get mixed. Evidence of postglacial human colonization dates back to 12000 years BC in Qinghai and 10000 years BC in Tibet have also been reported. It is thus possible that earliest domestication of yak was initiated by these colonizers as evidenced through 10000 years BC old yak remains in this area. Yak husbandry took a rapid growth in this area as archaeological records suggest several fold increase in abundance of yak products during 10000 to 5000 years BC. This growth was further aided by transition of vegetation from forests to steppe and alpine meadow in eastern Qinghai Tibetan Plateau during early Holocene age. Domesticated yak found outside China have originally descended from Chinese yak as evidenced by morphological data (Weiner *et al.*, 2003). From Qinghai and Tibet, yak spread rapidly to other parts of world. Domesticated yak migrated to the east, from the Bayan Kala Mountains into the Songpan grasslands and Danba mountains. To the south, the migration went through passes in the Himalayas to the mountainous grasslands of the southern slopes of the range. To the west, yak entered Kashmir through the western Tibet grasslands. And to the north the migration took the yak over the Kunlun Mountains into northern Pamir, northern and southern Tianshan and Altai. In all areas, their natural habitat range reside at altitude of 3000-5000 m with no or little trees and bushes and are interspersed with marshes, swamps and lakes.

2.4 Breeds of yak

Breed may be defined as the group of animals related by descent and having same characteristics like general appearance, features, size, configuration etc. There may be considerable differences among individuals; still they have a group of many common points which distinguish them from other group. Such a common group is termed as breed. The purity of the breed is maintained by confining the mating of animals to within the breed.

Eleven yak breeds were officially recognized by committees of yak experts on the basis of intensive investigations in the six main yak-raising provinces in China. Though, some authors reported the number as 14. The recognized breeds are the Jiulong yak and Maiwa yak in Sichuan, Tianzhu White yak and Gannan yak in Gansu, Pali yak, Jiali (Alpine) yak and Sibu yak in Tibet, Huanhu yak, Plateau yak in Qinghai, Bazhou yak in Xinjiang and Zhongdian yak in Yunnan. The long-hair-forehead yak of Qinghai province is not considered as a breed because of its random distribution in herds of both the Huanhu and Plateau yak. However, all 11 breeds are distinguished only by origin, location and some small differences in productive characteristics (which might be attributable to the region). There is almost no evidence available of the magnitude of any genetic differences.

However, differences in aspects such as body size and milk production, as well as reproductive performance, might converge in a common environment. Currently, genetic approaches using chromosomal and protein polymorphisms, mitochondrial DNA RFLP (restricted fragment length polymorphism), mitochondrial DNA sequencing and microsatellite genotyping are being introduced to the study of yak to estimate the genetic distance among breeds and some aspects of breed differentiation. The detailed characteristics of different breed are given below:

Plateau yak

This breed is found on the cold highland pasture of southern and northern Qinghai province where the wild yak distribution overlapped with it, particularly in historical times. Crossing between them is thus assumed to have taken place. Its population numbers around three million (Han Jianlin, 2000). The Plateau yak of Qinghai looks similar to the wild yak in body conformation. Among domestic yak breeds it stands tall, has a relatively large body weight with big head. Both sexes are horned. Similar to wild yak, it has greyish-white hair down its back and around the muzzle and eye sockets. It adapts well to the cold and humid climate at high elevation.

Huanhu yak

This breed is found in the transitional zone around the Qinghai Lake in Qinghai province where the grasslands are predominantly semi-arid and consist of meadow pasture. It is believed that herds of this strain were domesticated and transferred to this area by the Qiang people. The Huanhu yak, numbering about one million (Han Jianlin, 2000), contains some remnants of cattle blood from the time of its origins, and this may account for some of its differences from the Plateau yak. The Huanhu has a relatively smaller body size and finer structure, a wedge-shaped head, a narrower and longer nose that is mostly concave in the middle, a smaller but broad mouth, a thinner neck, deeper chest, narrower buttock, longer legs and smaller, but strong solid feet with a hard base to them as compared to Plateau yak. Most of the animals are hornless; those with horns have a fine, long and slightly curved set of horns. The colours are varied, but the majority is black-brown.

Tianzhu White yak

The Tianzhu White breed is found in patches of Gansu province, which is located in the eastern end of the Qilian mountains and the northern edge of the Qinghai-Tibetan Plateau. Its main distribution borders the Menyuan and Huzhu counties of Qinghai where a few white yak are also found. Generally, 2 - 3 percent of all yak populations are white individuals - though these are not regarded as part of the Tianzhu White breed. Because the white yak hair is easily dyed into different colours, it has been highly valued in local markets. Accordingly the farmers, who had migrated from Qinghai started to select and breed pure white herds about a century ago. The breed has a medium body size and fine structure, a well-developed forepart but a less-developed rear part and strong but short legs. And there are big differences in size between the two sexes. Compared to the females, the males have larger heads with a wider forehead, longer and coarser horns with a visible contour, a larger mouth and broader muzzle, thinner lips, smaller nose and a coarser neck.

Gannan yak

Gannan Yak is also found in Gansu province and the population is about 7,00,000 of this breed (Han Jianlin, 2000). It has a strong body conformation and well-developed muscles, a relatively large skull, a short, wide and slightly protruding forehead, a long and concave nose with externally expanded muzzle, a square mouth with thin lips. The animals may be horned (48 - 97 percent in different herds) or hornless with small ears, round eyes, a well-developed chest and belly and short, strong legs with small feet. Black is the predominant colour. The males have longer and coarser horns with wider distance between the bases and a stronger neck than the females. The females have a small udder with short nipples (Rongchang, 1989).

Pali yak

This breed is mainly found in Tibet which borders western Bhutan and India. It has a strong and well-developed body conformation that is rectangular, a short skull with a wide forehead, a big round mouth with thin lips, small eyes, broad muzzle, small nose, a short, strong neck, a deep wide chest and large heart girth, a large belly and short, strong legs with small solid feet. Most of the animals have horns with wide bases. Black is the dominant body colour.

Sibu yak

This breed is found in Lhasa, capital of Tibet. It has a large head with externally expanded horns, a rectangular-shaped body conformation with a straight back.

Jiali (Alpine) yak

This breed is also found in the Jiali part of Tibet at the southern edge of the Nyenchen Thangla mountains and the name follows as Jiali. It has a relatively large body shape with a deep and wide chest, and it is mostly horned. Compared to the females, males have coarser and stronger horns with a wide distance between the bases. Females have a thinner neck, straighter back, a larger belly and shorter legs than the males. Eighty percent of the animals have a white-spotted head or a completely white head.

Jiulong yak

This breed belongs to the Jiulong part of Sichuan province, which is located on the southeastern edge of the Qinghai-Tibetan Plateau. The population now numbers around 50 000 animals (Jincheng, 1996). The Jiulong yak has a large body height and body size, with a deep and wide chest and a medium-sized head. The breed is horned. Males, compared to females, have a shorter head but with a wider forehead and wider-based horns, bigger eyes, thinner lips and well-developed teeth, a finer neck, straighter back and shorter legs. Females have a relatively long neck. Black is the predominant colour (61.7 percent); the rest are black-and-white (24.6 percent).

Maiwa yak

Population of this breed is around 6,00,000 (Xiaowei and Guanghui, 1998) and mostly found in Sichuan province, which borders Gansu and Qinghai provinces. The breed originated from almost the same locality as the present-day Jiulong yak. However, it was taken by a migratory tribe to its present habitat, passing through southern Qinghai, perhaps in the 1st decade of nineteenth century. During that migration, perhaps mating occurred with other domestic yak on route and with wild yak when it first settled in Hongyuan, when wild yak were still known to come down from Qinghai. The resulting infusions of genes are thought to have improved the original type. The better pasture and ecological environment of the new habitat assisted its development. It has a medium-sized head and a wide flat forehead, straight back, a well-developed belly, a long body with short legs and small solid feet. Most of the animals are horned. Black accounts for 64.2 percent of the population, the rest are black with a white-spotted head and tail (Li, 1992).

Bazhou yak

This breed is found mainly in Xinjiang province. This breed has a large rectangular body, a heavy head, a short and wide forehead, big round eyes, small ears, a broad muzzle and thin lips, a wide chest, large belly and strong legs with small, solid feet. The majority (77.3 percent) have fine, long horns. Black is the main colour, but some are black and white, brown or grey and white (Rongchang, 1989).

Zhongdian yak

This breed is found in northern part of Yunnan province, at the southern end of the Qinghai-Tibetan Plateau where it borders Tibet and Sichuan. In general, the breed of yak has had frequent exchanges of blood with yak in Sichuan. There are about 20 000 animals of this breed (Jincheng, 1996). It has a strong body conformation, large round eyes, small ears, a wide forehead, a deep chest, straight back, well-developed legs with large feet and a short tail. Both sexes have horns. There is relatively large variation in body size. The majority of the animals are black (62.4 percent), a black-and-white colouring is found among 27.5 percent of them, while the rest are black with white-spots on the forehead, legs and tail (Rongchang, 1989).

Indian yak breeds

National Research Centre on Yak conducted survey in the last decade in India (Ramesha *et al.*, 2009) and reported that yak may be categorized in to 5 types i.e, Common, Bisonian, Bareback, Hairy forehead and White yaks. Common type yak are comparatively smaller in size and the appearance of the head and body conformation are like cattle. In India, around 60 percent yaks are common type. Bisonian type are hefty animals with compact head connected to the main trunk by strong and short neck, hairs on forehead curled and 30 percent of this type (Ramesha *et al.*,2008). The bareback type yaks have rectangular body with short hairs on rump and wither. The hairy forehead type has bushy hair on forehead which sometime covers the eye. Their color varies from ash, yellowish to black with white patches. White type, as indicated in the name, is white in colour and a rare type. Based on geographical area the Indian yak may be classified into Ladakh type, Arunachal yaks, Himachal yaks and Sikkim yaks.

Ladakh yaks

Yak in this region may be of three type viz., Feral, Mountain and Plateau (Gupta and Kumar,1994). Feral yaks are large size, weighing more than 500 kg and they have angular body covered with long, coarse and glossy hair on body as well as on tail with an undercoat of mohair. Mountain type is found in high altitude of Ladakh characterized by massive body, angular body and bisonian horns. Body is mostly of solid black or brown with long fringe which sometime touches the ground. Plateau type is of medium size, weighing around 250-400 kg and is similar to cattle in their body conformation. These are found in lower altitudes and crossing with cattle occurs due to intermixing of herds in grazing, banks of stream.

Arunachal yaks

These vary in their body conformation and other phenotypic characters. Yaks in West Kemong district resembles with the Bhutan yaks while Tawang region is similar to those with Eastern Tibet (Nivsarkar *et al.*, 1997).

Sikkim yaks

Nivsarkar *et al.* (1997) classified the Sikkim yaks into two: Bho and Aho type depending on the geographical distribution and community rear them in the state.

Himachal yak

Lahul & Spiti valley and Pangi valley have the yak population, though in less numbers as compared to other states or region. These are very sturdy and massive similar to yaks of mountain type found in Ladakh region. Sangla valleys have also few yaks but are smaller in size and are compact.

2.5 Distribution

Yak lives predominantly on the high altitude areas of China, Mongolia, India and Pakistan. The centre of the yak's distribution is the Qinghai-Tibetan Plateau, which is interspersed with several mountain ranges. The place extends over 2.5 million sq km and was described by Miller (1995) as the most extensive high-elevation region on earth and the low quality grazing lands. These areas are, to a large extent, above the tree line where there is virtually no or little cropping. At its high elevation, the territory overall is characterized by a harsh climate of cool summers, severely cold winters and grazing resources restricted by very short growing seasons.

Yak are found extensively on the plateau of alpine and subalpine regions at altitudes from 2 000 - 5 000 m with a cold, arid and harsh climate. The area extends from the southern slopes of the Himalayas in the south to the Altai in the north and from the Pamir in the west to the Minshan mountains in the east. From the most recently available information, the number of yak in Chinese territories is estimated to exceed 13 million, of which about 15 percent are hybrids with (mostly) *Bos taurus* cattle of local types. The majority of the yak in India, as shown in Table 1, is in Jammu and Kashmir followed by Arunachal Pradesh. The rest of the world accounts for another million or so yak. The yak of Nepal and Bhutan are on the southern slopes of the Himalayas while those of India are distributed in the high altitude northern provinces and in the small territory of Sikkim. Other pockets of yak populations are in alpine areas of Afghanistan and Pakistan, adjacent to the Qinghai-Tibetan Plateau of China. Its imperative to indicate that, Ladakh

Province of Jammu & Kashmir comprising around 26,000 yak population but decreasing day by day due to mechanization in agriculture and transport system. In India, few states have only yak population and the statewise population is shown in the following table.

Table 2.1 : State-wise yak population in India

S. no	State	Population
1	Arunachal Pradesh	14,000
2	Jammu & Kashmir	62,000
3	Himachal Pradesh	2,000
4	Uttaranchal	500
5	West Bengal	300
6	Sikkim	5,000
Total		83, 800

Source: Basic Animal Husbandry Statistics, Dept of Animal Husbandry, Dairying & Fisheries, Ministry of Agriculture, Govt of India, New Delhi

References

Flerow, C.C. 1980. On the geographic distribution of the genus Poephagus during the Pleistocene and Holocene. *Quaternary Paleontol. (East) Berlin*, 4: 123-126.

Gatesy J., Amato G., Vrba E., Schaller G. and DeSalle R. 1997. A cladistic analysis of Mitochondrial ribosomal DNA from the Bovidae. *Molecular Phylogenetics and Evolution* 7(3):703–719.

Guo, S, Savolainen,P, Su,J, Zhang,Q, Qi, D,Zhou, J, Zhong,Y,Zhano,X and Liu, J. 2006.Origin of mitochondrial DNA diversity of domestic yaks. BMC Evolutionary Biology. 6: 73-85.

Gupta S.C and Kumar, P. Technical Report on visit to Livestock Genetic Resources of Ladakh. NBAGR (ICAR). Karnal, Haryana.

Han Jianlin 2000. Conservation of yak genetic diversity in the Hindu Kush Himalayan region and central Asian steppes. *In* Shrestha, J.N.B. (ed), *Proceedings of the fourth global conference on conservation of domestic animal genetic resources, in Kathmandu, 17-21 August 1998*. pp. 113-116.

Jincheng, Z. 1996. *Yak genetics and breeding*. Chengdu, China, Sichuan Scientific and Technology Press. 271 pp.

Lenstra J.A. and Bradley D.G. 1999. Systematics and phylogeny of cattle. In: Fries R. and Ruvinsky A. (eds), *Genetics of Cattle*. CAB (Commonwealth Agricultural Bureau) International, Wallingford, Oxon, UK. pp. 1–14.

Li, C. 1992. *China yak*. Beijing, China Agriculture Press. 254 pp.

Miller, D.J. (1995). Herds on the Move: Winds of change among pastoralists in the Himalayas and on the Tibetan Plateau. ICIMOD, Kathmandu, Nepal.

Nivsarkar, A.E., Gupta, S.C. and Gupta, N. 1997.Yak production . Directorate of Publication and Information on ICAR. New Delhi.pp- 393.

Ramesha, K.P., Biswas, T.K., Kataktalware,M.A. 2008. Breeding strategies for genetic improvement of Indian yaks. Livestock International. 12: 14-17.

Ramesha,K.P.,Biswas, T.K. and Jayakumar,S. 2009. Status and strategies for genetic improvement of Indian yaks in high reaches of the Himalayas. Proc. On International Conference on yak husbandry- challenges and strategies. National Research Centre on Yak, Dirang, Arunachal Pradesh. Pp- 10-16.

Rongchang, Z. 1989. *China: the yak*. Lanzhou, China, Gansu Scientific and Technology Press. 386 pp.

Rongchang, Z. 1989. *China: the yak*. Lanzhou, China, Gansu Scientific and Technology Press. 386 pp.

Wiener,G., Jianlin,H and Ruijun,L. 2003. The Yak.2nd Edition. The Regional Office for Asia and Pacific, Food and Agricultural Organization of the United Nations. Bangkok, Thailand. Pp- 1-44.

Xiaowei, L. and Guanghui, Z. 1998. Present situation and development strategy of yak husbandry in Sichuan. *Forage and Livestock*, Supplement: 26-28.

□□□

Chapter 3

Adaptation to Cold Climate

3.1. Introduction

Adaptation is a term used to describe the ways in which organisms change over time in response to the changing demands of their environment. Organisms seem to accumulate certain physiological, behavioral, and structural traits gradually, and these traits aid them in their ability to survive and reproduce under existing environmental conditions.

Adaptation is a long term and complex phenomenon and needs alteration of complex biological processes that need several hundreds of years. The capacity to survive must be one of the most important traits in the genetic make up of the yaks. The yak is one of the rarest animal species which not only survives and reproduces normally in extremely harsh environment at high altitude but has also been providing the basic subsistence to man living there for centuries.

Yaks are predominantly found at altitude ranging from 2000 to 6000 meters which is cold and semi-humid throughout the year.

Sometimes, they found at an altitude of 7200 meters, where they play an important role in the transportation of goods. In winter, temperature reaches to as low as -40°C, even in sometimes reaches to -50°C. In summer, average temperature varies between 4°C-6°C. Average relative humidity remains between 50 to 65%. The yak is a specialized species that has adapted to living in these harsh and high altitude environments, where other bovines will not survive, or at least, not thrive. The yak thrives at cold high altitude, reproduces and produces milk, meat, wool and other products to fulfill various socio-cultural functions within the pastoral society. Majority of the world yaks are found in China and Mongolia. Rests of the yak population are distributed to other countries like Kazakhstan, Tajikistan, Tuva, Buryat, Russia, Pakistan, Nepal, Bhutan and India. In India, they are found in Ladakh and Doda of Jammu and Kashmir, Kinnaur, Lahul sptiti and Pangi of Himachal Pradesh, Uttarkashi and Pithoragarh of Uttarakhand, North, East and West districts of Sikkim and Twang and West Kameng districts of Arunachal Pradesh. Various metaphorical expressions for the domestic yak emphasize its importance for transportation of goods and services throughout western Asia: *"ship of the cold region"*, *"biological snow plough"* and *"boat of the plateau"*.

Yaks live in the extremely harsh climatic conditions along with various kinds of stresses which are not very much favourable for life. The stresses are discussed below:

a) Extreme cold throughout the year

Yaks are well adapted to the extreme cold climatic condition at the very high altitude where average annual temperature varies between -3°C to +3°C. Winter temperatures is as low as -40°C. Even at this low temperature yak can freely move on the grassland and take feed. The lower temperature which can be tolerated by the yak is not finding out.

b) Low O_2 as well as atmospheric pressure

With the increased altitude atmospheric pressure as well as O_2 pressures both decreases constantly. Atmospheric pressure at the elevation about 4000m (468 mmHg) decreases to 61% than the sea level (760 mmHg) and it become 52% at the elevation about 5000m (398 mmHg). The reduced P_{O2} at high altitude results in reduced oxygen loading in the lungs such that the blood may not carry a sufficient supply of oxygen to the cells of respiring tissues. The lower atmospheric pressure along with lower O_2 pressure imposes threat to the life of the yak. However, they can cope up it efficiently by various adaptive mechanisms.

c) High solar radiation

At the altitude where yak population mostly found, the average annual sunshine remains about 2000 hours, whereas the same at sea level is over 3000 hours. However, as per solar radiation is concern, it remains very high at high altitute in comparison to the sea level. At very high altitude the level of annual solar radiation ranges between 130 and 165 Kcal/cm^2 (540-690 KJ/cm^2). However, at sea level, annual solar radiation vary around 40-50 kcal/cm^2. High solar radiation may cause severe damage to the skin and may damage other important functions of the body.

d) High altitude and sloppy mountainous terrain

Yak can comfortably live with the altitude of 5500 meters. Reports suggest that yak steer used as pack animals are capable of traversing terrain at 7200 meters. Along with high altitude, sloppy mountain terrain always foist to the life of the yak. Any careless move to the steep slope can cause the end of the life of the yak.

e) Limited herbage growing period and wide variety of herbage sparely distributed

Major constrain to the life of the yak is the severe shortage of feed and fodder at high altitude. The yaks have to suffer from inadequate feeding under the traditional farming system, resulting in big seasonal body weight variations, low milk production, and low fertility. The saying that yaks are "alive in summer, strong in autumn, thin in winter, and tired in spring" is an accurate description of yaks. Natural feeds are available for the animals are grass, sedges (wet land plants) and forbs (broad leaved herbicious plants). Due to the freezing temperature maximum part of the year, average herbage growing period remain 4 to 6 months in most of the yak raising areas. Except herbage growing period, the ground is covered with thick snow, therefore shortage of feed is acute and intense especially in the winter season. Yaks are capable of not only surviving but also working by consuming the broken and wilted blades of grass. They can remain even without food for several days during snowing without any appreciable adverse effect on their health. Even when poor food is available, yaks can carry their load 15 to 17 km in a day and stay in good condition.

All these stresses are interrelated. Altitude and air temperature are related as are annual precipitation and annual sunshine. All these factors have an effect on the growth and type of the herbage in the area and thus, availability of the herbage for the yak.

3.2. Adaptive mechanisms

The above mentioned various types of stresses create unfavourable environment for the subsistence of the animals. Among which very low temperature is the major one. Unlike natural phenomenon, yak sustains in cold climate through conserving heat, rather than generating heat. Heat generation requires feed which is not available abundantly in major cases. However, yaks make it possible to survive, produce and reproduce in this miserable climatic condition by developing various adaptive mechanisms. The adaptive mechanisms are classified into major five categories which are enlisted below:

1. Anatomical/structural adaptation
2. Physiological adaptation
3. Behavioural adaptation
4. Reproductive adaptation
5. Metabolic adaptation

3.2.1. Anatomical/structural adaptation

a) Compact body

Yak's body is compact. Large body mass incomparison to the body surface area helps less dissipation of heat from the body as less area is exposed to the harsh environment. Surface area is about 0.016 m^2/kg body weight which is much less compare to the cattle.

b) Small body parts (appendages)

Protruding body parts of the yak are short or small e.g., short neck, small ears, no dewlap and short tail. As the body parts are comparatively smaller, the surface area exposed the environment is also limited. About 40-42% short limbs compare to the local cattle is another remarkable feature of the yak. Small and hairy udder along with short teats (2.5-4 cm) is covered with thick fine hair of the yak cows ensures protection from the chilled weather and maintain normal milk production. Frostbite is not usually observed in any part of the body.

c) Strong limbs and small hooves

Yak is known as the "ships of the plateau". Yaks are highly valued for their sure-footed capabilities in packing large loads over long distances even in a potentially dangerous situation, such as marshy ground. They are safer than horses for riding in swampy ground, through rivers or on steep rocky slopes. Long legs have strong small hooves of compact texture with a narrow and sharp hoof tip, hard hoof edges and a close hoof fork, and pseudo-claws. There is an area of soft cutis on the sole. These structures serve as support when the animal wanders on the high mountains with precipitous terrain. The forelegs are short but as thick and strong as the hindlegs. Strong legs and hoof structure helps them to walk smoothly in the steep rocky slopes. The hoofs are small and compact texture, with a narrow and sharp hoof tip, hard hoof edges and a close hoof fork. These typical hoof characteristics make deep imprints on the ground, and may be an adaptation to allow the yak to control its movement when going downhill as movement towards downhill in a steep slope is very difficult task.

d) Skin

i. *Skin thickness* : Very small number of skin wrinkles on the body surface of the yak giving the animal a relatively small radiation surface. The yak skin is thick, unwrinkled along with well developed dermal layer and fat layer compared to the different breeds of the cattle. Average skin thickness (mm) of yak, *Bos taurus* and *Bos indicus* are 6.20, 6.12 and 5.62, respectively. Within the body back portion has the thickest skin as back portion of the yaks are mostly exposed to the chilly wind, rain and snow. Average skin thickness (mm) in the shoulder blade, back and knee are 5.60±0.36, 7.50±0.83 and 5.60±0.40, respectively.

ii. *Sweat glands density and secretion* : Like cattle, sweat gland of the yak is apocrine type with long and tortuous ductules distributed in the skin throughout the body. Sweat glands are mostly non-functional. However, only muzzle has some functional sweat gland and which can secrete sweat. Highest sweat gland density is reported in the forehead (891/cm^2) and lowest density is reported in the rump (138/cm^2) with an overall average density of 399±251/cm^2. Non-functional sweat glands help to preserve the heat through the prevention of evaporative heat loss. These helps to succeed yak heat tolerant, but make yak intolerant to heat.

iii. *Subcutaneous fat* : A thick subcutaneous layer of fat provides insulation to the yak. Fat deposition normally occurs in the summer and early autumn when herbage growth is ample in the pasture. Besides insulation, subcutaneous fat also act as energy reserve to be utilised during energy deprivation especially in winter and early spring. In the young animals subcutaneous fat remains at low level, however as the animals grow into adult deposition of subcutaneous fat become increases.

iv. *Pigmented skin* : The skin of the yak is highly pigmented. Pigmented granules are abundantly found in the epidermis layer of the yak skin, especially in the cells of *stratum basale*. This attributes help to resist the effect of ultraviolet rays of solar radiation and subsequent injury to the deeper layer of the skin.

e) Hair coat

The thick hair coat is composed of long thick outer coarse hair, intermediate down fibers and short fine layer of down hairs, they are tangled together. The diameter of the outer coarse hair, intermediate down fibers and for fine down hair are about 52μ, 25–52μ and 25μ, respectively. Shaggy fringes of coarse hair cover the chest, shoulder, thighs and lower half of the tail, and hangs from the flank region of the yak. The hairs form bushy tuft between its horn and a great mane on its neck. Hair of the yak forehead is well developed can cover the eyes. Yak with white faces usually have eyes surrounded by black hair. These black hairs may protect the eyes the yak from exposure to solar radiation.

Thick hair coat of the yak not only act as insulator, but also protect the animals at high altitude from harmful ultraviolet rays. Thick hair coat especially the outer coarse hairs also guard the yak from the wet condition as coat has low water absorption capacity. The *erectores pilorum* muscles in the dermis of the yak are well developed and which contracts during heavy cold. Contraction of the muscles helps to increase the depth of fibre and thereby, trap more air which provides insulation. Inner down hairs provides additional insulation during intense cold condition.

The most notable feature of the yak adaptation against frozen cold is through the creation of opposite electrical charge between outer coarse hair and down hairs. The outer coarse hairs become negatively charged and inner down hairs become positively charged. During heavy snowstorm the charge difference enhances and thus hairs pack closure.

Above mentioned facts indicates that outer coarse hairs of yak safeguard against wetness, thus makes 'water proof' and inner down hairs along with outer coarse hairs protect against cold thus make the yak 'cold proof'. Therefore, coat of the yak play important role to survive in the prevailing weather condition at high altitude which conserve the body heat. In yak conservation of heat precedence over the generation of heat which require additional feed which is in short supply especially in winter.

Seasonal variation of coat composition : The growth of the down hairs is cyclical. The down hair follicles remain dormant during summer season. Just before winter, when the environmental temperature starts decline down hair follicles become active and down hairs grow densely especially in the shoulder, back and rump. The proportion of down hair may increase as high as 30%. Density of down fiber can be as high as about $3{,}000/cm^2$. However the outer coarse hair growth is not that much. Therefore, proportion of the outer coarse hair is decreased in the hair coat. With the increase of environmental temperature the down hairs starts shedding and its proportion in the hair coat reaches to the lowest at summer.

Variation of coat composition with the age : In the calfhood of the yak below six months of age the coat is composed of almost entirely down hairs. With the advancement of age, the proportion of down hairs decreases. The proportion (by weight) of down hairs reaches to 63% at one year old, 52% at two years old, 44% at three years old and 43% at four and five years old.

Colour of the hair coat : Yak hair colour usually varies from black and brown through variegation to white. In northern latitude where solar radiation is not so intense like southern latitude, white coloured yaks are mostly found and in southern latitude black and brown yaks are mostly found. Black or dark hairs absorb the radiation and convert into heat. The heat then transferred to skin by conduction down the hairs or through the still air trapped within the fur.

f) Mouth

Yak has broad mouths, small muzzles and thin flexible lips. The front (incisor) teeth are hard and broad and have a flat grinding surface. The tip of the tongue is broad and blunt. The surface of the tongue feels rough and "thorny". Their specialized tongue, covered with small thorny tubercles, allow them to easily lick up low-lying forages and incisor teeth and lips helps in creeping stems, and roots of grass. Typical structure of the mouth of the yak helps to graze on alpine sedges, grasses, forbs, lichens and mosses. Large nostrils of the yak support more air intake.

g) Trachea

At high altitude the animals need to inhale higher amount of air at faster rate to compensate the low O_2 tension. Compared to common cattle, yaks have a shorter and wider trachea to allow a high rate of air intake. The trachea of the yak is comparable with the dog. The length of trachea of white Yaks is about 44 - 51 cm (65 cm for other cattle at the same age), but the diameter is appreciably greater. Cross section of trachea found to be crescent shaped compared to the round shape in common cattle. A large space exists between the two ends of annular cartilage, being 5 cm in the adult male and 2.2 - 3 cm in the female yak. This type of tracheal structure allows yaks to breathe rapidly and to quickly increase air intake into the lungs when conditions demand it.

h) Chest

Yaks have 47 - 48 vertebrae, of which 14 - 15 are thoracic vertebrae and 14 pairs of ribs, one or two more than in other cattle. Ribs are long and narrow. In comparison to cattle the distance between ribs are large. This gives the yak larger chest capacities compare to the local cattle. Larger thorax and chest allow the development and accommodate large lungs and a large heart.

i) Large heart and lungs

At high altitude O_2 tension is low, thus capacity of the heart as well as lung should be well developed as well as sufficiently large enough to cope up the situation. Higher capacity lung will provide more surface area to absorb more O_2 to compensate the low O_2 tension. In yak the heart and lungs indexes (the ratio of heart and lung weight to body weight) are higher than in common cattle. Female yak has comparatively higher heart and lung index compare to male counterpart. The heart index is 0.52% and 0.42% in female and male yak respectively and the lung index is 0.98% and 0.75%, respectively in male and female yak. Cross section of lungs indicated that alveolar areas comprise about 59% of the lung compared to 40% in cattle. Right ventricle of the heart of yak is relatively larger and higher capilarisation compared to right ventricle which provide support to send oxygen-poor blood to the lungs.

j) Small udder covered with hairs

In female yak the udder is small and covered with hair. Smaller udder helps to the less exposure of the udder surface area to the cold environment and hair provides insulation to the udder.

k) Large size rumen

Rumen of yak was better developed than that of the cattle, based on the proportion of the weight of different parts to the total stomach. Relative percentages of the rumen and omasum of the domestic yak are about 50% larger and 200% smaller, respectively, than in some domestic cattle. A large rumen may be a useful adaptation to forage roughage achieved by natural selection under the particularly rough grazing conditions prevailing in the yak territories. The large rumen volume of yak relative to body size may be a useful adaptation to foraging herbage under rough grazing conditions.

3.2.2. Physiological adaptation

Physiological adaptation is an important aspect of the yak's adaptation to high altitude with scarce feed resources. Following are the adaptation skill developed by the yak over the years.

a) Presence of brown adipose tissue (BAT)

Brown adipose tissue (BAT) or brown fat is one of two types of fat or adipose tissue (the other being white adipose tissue) found in mammals. New born animals usually have abundant brown fat. Approximately 2% of the body weight of new-born calves appears to be brown adipose tissue. Primary function is to generate body heat in animals or newborns that do not shiver. The brown adipose tissue changed progressively to that of white adipose tissue as the age of the calves increased. Thus there is a gradual disappearance of brown fat stores within the first year of life as the mechanisms of themogenesis convert from non-shivering to shivering. In adult yak, higher amount of brown adipose tissue present around heart, kidney and tail, which provide heat during intense cold.

b) Respiration and heart rate

Highly variable respiration rate is reported in yak. At an ambient temperature of below 13°C respiration rate ranges between 20 and 30 per minute. As the temperature increases, the respiration rate rises rapidly. Diurnal variation of respiration rate is reported with a higher respiration rate in the evening than in the morning. During activity the respiration rate is higher than at the time of inactivity. However, respiration rate does not show significant change with humidity, wind speed or the prevailing weather. Reports suggested that the change of respiration rate not only due to the change of oxygen demand but also to regulate body temperature.

Heart rate is 45 - 79 times per minute and faster than in common cattle. However, lowest pulse rate is observed in the month of March when yak in their poorest condition and usually at a point of exhaustion. The condition occurs due to prolonged shortage of feed throughout the winter months leads to near to starvation condition and thus reduced metabolic rate.

c) Red blood cell and Myoglobin

At high-altitude due to lower partial oxygen pressure in the blood results into (40-60%) increase number of erythrocytes and in the production of haemoglobin to help offset the deficiency of oxygen to the tissue. However, yaks do not have exceptionally high concentration of erythrocytes in blood. The diameter of erythrocytes in yaks is larger than in common cattle, thus erythrocyte has greater surface area and higher oxygen retention capacity. The diameter of red blood cells in adult yaks was reported to be 4.83 µm, while that of local cattle was 4.38 ìm. Yaks generally have hemoglobins with higher oxygen binding affinities than those of their lowland relatives. Higher oxygen carrying capacity of the yak's erythrocytes helps to adapt at high altitude.

d) Diffusion capacity of lungs

The alveolar area occupies about 59 percent of the cross-sectional area of the yak lungs, compared with 40 percent for local cattle. Thus, Yak lungs provides larger surface area over the pulmonary membrane and ultimately higher diffusing capacity for oxygen in order to compensate for the lower oxygen content of the air. During respiration, the lung volume in yak is greatly increased which expands the surface area of the alveolar membrane to facilitate oxygen diffusion.

e) Reduce vasoconstrictor reflex

Lower atmospheric pressure at high altitudes inhibits diffusion of oxygen from the air into the lungs and creates chronic hypoxic condition. Vasoconstriction commonly occurs in order to reduce blood supply to under- ventilated areas of the lung. At high altitude, such vasoconstriction would not be a good long term response to permanently hypoxic conditions because the whole lung becomes a low-oxygenated area at high altitude, the vasoconstriction reflex would be very damaging, as it would then affect the whole lung. Yak has successfully adapted to chronic hypoxia with the attenuation of the hypoxic pulmonary vasoconstrictor response, associated genetic adaptations to hypoxia. However, cows although in the same genus can not sustain chronic hypoxic condition.

f) Post natal presence of foetal haemoglobin

Newborn's blood has four types of hemoglobin. Foetal type of hemoglobin (HbF1 and HbF2) represents 49% and adult type hemoglobin (HbI and HbII) represent about 51% of total hemoglobin. Foetal haemoglobin has higher affinity of the oxygen than the adult haemoglobin. Foetal haemoglobin especially HbF2 (although present only about 8.9% of the total hemoglobin) has higher affinity for oxygen and plays an important role in the survival of yak neonates in low oxygen environments. There are about 41-100% one type foetal haemoglobin present at the time of birth in calves (cattle). However, it's proportion decreases rapidly after birth and totally replaced by adult haemoglobin at 2-3 months of age.

g) Cellular acclimatization

In animals native to altitudes of 13,000 to 17,000 ft mitochondria and cellular oxidative enzyme system are slightly more plentiful than in sea level counterparts which cause more efficient utilization of oxygen in those high altitude living animals. Therefore, it is presumed that same mechanisms may hold good in yak too.

h) Less urination and excretion

The number of glomeruli present in the kidney is less in comparison the animals are in plain. Therefore, excretion of urine as well as excreta is less which helps in maintaining water balance in the body.

i) Loss of body weight in winter

The growth rate of yak generally is not constant. Body weight fluctuates significantly by season throughout the life. The body weight decrease in the cold season is followed by a large increase (compensatory growth) during the warm season. The weight loss of calves over the first winter was around 12-15 percent of the weight before the onset of winter. Typically, over the following summer and autumn, young yak regain their weight losses and may gain double in weight before again losing, over the second winter of life, perhaps 25 percent of the maximum weight reached. The cycle of weight gain and weight loss continues throughout life. In fully adult yak, the weight loss in the cold season is roughly equal to the gain in the following warm season. These cyclical changes of body weight is due to the annual nutrient supply of grassland varies greatly with the season. Yak can survive even after huge body weight loss during winter. This type of phenomenon is essential for their survival in their normal habitat.

j) Peculiarities in lactation

In extreme winter when lactating yak starts loosing body weight due to severe shortage of feeds and severe cold, even then the female yaks can produce little amount of milk for her calf. In the very next year summer season (i.e., second year of calving), the female yak again starts giving milk, provided the yak female do not conceive. Their milk yield is about 1/2 or 1/3rd to that in the first year of calving and also peak milk production in the month of July and August. These females are called "half-lactation cows" by local people. This is a unique lactation phenomenon among yak. On the other hand, lactating yaks in the year of calving are normally called "full-lactation cows". Yak does not dry off when milking ceases at the end of the warm season, and the calf, when present, continues to take some milk. The mammary gland of half-lactating yaks maintained an active secreting state, although it has undergone a longer period of lactation than yaks at late lactation. The reduced milk yield in the half lactating yaks might be caused by the normal involution of mammary gland, similar to cows prior to entering the dry period and again rejuvenate in the next summer when sufficient feeds and fodders are available.

3.2.3. Behavioural adaptation

Kind of behaviour developed in yak which helps them to survive and produce in their natural habitat. Behaviourally, the yak is active and easily excited and can have a ferocious temper. Its conditioned reflexes make it respond rapidly to danger and external forces. In the grazing situation, yak will often jump and run, pursuing each other with tail in the air. Yak can also roll over on pastures as horses do - but unlike other bovines.

They prefer to stay out of the wind during the coldest days or will face into the wind as their long thick forehead and front quarter hair is thicker there than on the backside. In the hot days of summer, the yak retreat to the cool barn or find shade and reduce activity until the cooler afternoon or evening when they get fired up and have to "get it out of their system".

a) Herding tendency

Yaks are herding ungulates. They are very gregarious. They prefer to stay in group and therefore form large herds for protection, particularly against wolves, but they are also nervous of wild animals and man and, if startled, will readily take flight. Groups are not stable through time. Grouping behavior depends on sex, time of year, and location. Group types included solitary adult males, mixed-aged males, females and offspring, and mixed sexes; females rarely occur alone or in groups of <5–10 individuals.

b) Easily tamed and trained

Yak usually grazes round the year. They neither require elaborate housing, nor usually fenced in or tethered, except at the time of milking. Yak has the ability to be readily trained. Thus, they are easily trained to return to the campsite by the call of their names, or by special cries or singing. Yak finds their way back to the campsite without a herder - if it is not too far away. Yak are also readily tamed and trained for use as pack animals or for riding. Once trained, yak retains their acquired behaviour for a long time.

c) Migration

Migratory behaviour of the yak is very much important for their survival in the harsh climate. Typically they moves up and down slopes seasonally to take advantage of the best forage availability. The migration may vary from region to region, depending on the local availability of forages, seasonal temperature etc. During summer month yak migrate from lower elevation to the higher elevation i.e., near to snowline. Again in winter, they return back to the lower elevation. Yaks are well insulated and tolerate cold temperatures better than summer heat, and their movements reflect this preference.

d) Grazing behaviour

Yaks graze over variety of plant species available (alpine sedges, grasses, forbs, lichens and mosses) in the high altitude. Yak can graze long grass using their tongues, as is common for cattle, but they can also graze very short herbage, as is the case of sheep, by using their incisor teeth and lips. Yaks also graze rapidly and for long hours. Under most normal conditions, yaks have learned to avoid poisonous or thorny plants as recorded instances of poisoning are very rare.

Intake time : Total intake time depends upon the season, pasture condition, quality of pasture, structure of the yak herd in terms of sex and age. Usually intake time varies between 34-80 percent of the total available time for grazing. Rest of the time is used for walking, resting and drinking. Lactating females usually spend more time in grazing due to the higher demand of nutrient. The females have young calves at foot, and then grazing time is increased due to disturbance in grazing by the calf, frequently suckle.

In alpine pasture, the weather condition may become hostile in any moment. Yaks have adapted to consume maximum amount of grasses in a shortest possible time. Therefore, bite of the yak is quicker and nearer to the ground than that of any other species of cattle.

Distance traveled : The speed of movement in the pasture depends upon the season and pasture condition. At the start of the day, yak move fast than later on. Due to space vegetation in winter months, the movement is rapid than summer season. During summer they consume about 35 kg of herbages whereas in winter the values may come down to about 13 kg. In extreme winter, when ground is covered with snow and ice, yaks break through the cover to the wilted grass beneath, using their hooves and heads. Although severe scarcity of vegetation at high altitude deserts, still yak can get their feed until the snow is soft and not deeper than 10-12 cm.

Though, grazing yak meet the energy and protein requirement for maintenance, work and production, but in the later parts of the winter and the early spring they fall below the requirements. Yak then lose weight and condition.

Night grazing : Night grazing in yak is common during summer months. During hot periods of the day time they take rest and ruminate, prefer to graze at the cooler part of the day and if required at night.

Close grazing : Yak has strong prehensile tongue which helps to take long grasses like cattle. When the availability of grasses is limited or not available then it can graze over the short grass and creeping stems, and roots of grass. As yak has strong incisor teeth and lips, they can graze close to the ground as sheep do.

e) Rumination behaviour

In summer months, usually pasture is well developed and availability of herbages is higher. Then, yaks have four periods of rumination each day. The first period of rumination is generally two hours after the start of morning grazing. A second period is around noon, when the ambient temperature is high and yak stop grazing. A third period of rumination occurs about two hours before the animals are driven from the pasture back to the campsite. A fourth period is in the evening. Rumination periods generally last between 0.8 and 1.9 hours. Occasionally yaks ruminate at night, but usually they lie in a state of light sleep. Frequency of contractions of the rumen reticulum is similar at resting and grazing whereas in cattle it is only half at the time of resting or rumination.

f) Sure-footedness

Sure-footedness means skilled and confident in moving and so unlikely to stumble or fall. At very high altitude, where yak mostly found, the territories marked by steep, treacherous slopes, moor land, bogs and lakes. Animals like sheep or horse can not reach to that place; however, yak can reach and cope well in the marshy ground as they are sure-footed animal. Yak has strong limbs and small hooves of compact texture, with a narrow and sharp hoof tip, hard hoof edges and a close hoof fork. Typical hoof structure makes deep imprints in the ground which allow the yak to control its momentum when going downhill and move freely in difficult, precipitous terrain. In marshy land there is always a chance of sinking. In case of danger of sinking, yak will spread out their legs and use the underside of their bodies to prevent them from sinking. They will plod on with a swimming-kind of motion rather than panic and thrash around as a horse might. Yaks are well swimmer and they are well at trekking through snow. They can even be used to make tracks through the snow to clear paths for people - a sort of "biological snow plough".

3.2.4. Reproductive adaptation

In the harsh environmental condition, the existence of a species solely depends upon the maintenance of adequate level of reproduction. In general yak is reproductively poor calving relatively late for the first time and not regularly thereafter. Last stage of pregnancy is coincide severe shortage of feed over several months. The lack of sufficient feed over winter leads to loss of weight and body condition, both often severe, in the female yak. Still yak reproduce itself in this adverse conditions.

a) Seasonal breeder

Successful breeding takes place during the favourable season of the year i.e., in the summer months. Favourable temperature along with feed availability favours towards successful reproduction. Calf born early in the summer and get proper feed before reaching to the harsh winter season when availability of feed and fodder is least along with severe cold. Therefore, seasonal breeding helps survival of the calves from the harsh climatic condition.

b) Longer oestrus period

Yaks are graze through out the day and travel long distance for grazing. To achieve higher reproductive rate, oesturs or heat period of yak is comparatively higher in comparison to cattle. In a particular year, number of oestrous cycle is limited as they are seasonal breeder. As heat period is longer, chance of mating in a particular oestrus phase is higher. Oestrus in yak cows lasts for 2-4 days with an overall range of 10 to 118 hours; in some cases it may last for 5-7 or 8-9 days.

c) Short gestation period

Gestation period of yak is about 258 days and about one month shorter than cattle. Short gestation, with consequently smaller calves, leads to a less stressful and quicker parturition, a lower oxygen requirement by the calf and less body-weight loss by the cow. The shorter gestation period may benefit the female by reducing the load on the heart and respiratory system. The shorter gestation period and lower weight of newborn calves are a result of the adaptation of yaks to their habitat.

d) Nearly effortless parturition process

As the size of calf is small, the process of parturition remains nearly stress-less and quicker. Very rare case of dystokia is reported. Parturition of the domestic yak occurs during the day, rarely at night, in a sheltered location away from the herd. Birth is often from a standing position although the female may spend considerable time lying on her side. Calving takes place mainly in spring (from March to May) at pasture without any intervention by man.

e) Small, compact scrotum covered with hairs

Semen production necessitates optimum temperature, just below the body temperature. Excessive chilling condition may hamper the semen production. The scrotum of the male yak is small, compact and cover with hair. Smaller and compact size of the scrotum provides less exposure of scrotal surface area to the extreme cold climatic condition. Thicker cover of hair provides insulation to the scrotum. Thus, ensures normal sperm production.

f) Miniature calves

Newborn yaks are smaller (10 to 16 kg) than new born cattle calves both absolutely and relatively. Usually the weight of newborn cattle calves varies from 6.5 to 8% of the adults weight while weight of a newborn yaks ranges between 3 to 7 % of adult weight. The relatively low birth weight is a consequence of a relatively short gestation length (average 258 days) and that the fact that in mid- and late pregnancy the yak, typically, has to exist on ground that is frozen and covered with ice and snow. Also, the yak does not normally have the benefit of supplementary feeding. Due to nutritional deficiency, the physical condition of the female yak is at its lowest in late pregnancy. This condition leads to nutrient deficiency for the foetus at the very time when the foetus is at its most demanding. These condition favours miniature calves for the sustainability in the harsh environment.

3.2.5. Metabolic adaptation

Constant heat production irrespective of altitude is essential for the survival of the animals. Irrespective of altitude, fasting heat production of yak remains constant in contrast to cattle. Yak has the unique capability to conserve heat at cold temperatures, rather than by generating it, which would require food that may not be abundant. The fasting heat production (FHP) in the yak seems low compared with those of other species. The significant reduction of FHP in the winter may be due either to an altitude–temperature interaction or to the anatomical and physiological adaptation of the yak to the cold, or to both. The lower metabolic rate near the thermoneutral range (8–14°C), and its absence in response to increase of altitude, may be related to the species characteristics well adapted to the low O_2 concentration, extremely cold environment and long-term under-nutrition in the Tibet plateau or trans himalayan range.

Adaptation of yak at very high altitude plays tremendous role for their survival, produce and reproduce. Above mentioned adaptive mechanisms are helpful to cope various kind and level of stresses.

❑❑❑

Chapter 4

Reproduction

The yak (*Bos grunniens*) is an amazing animal that inhabits in their natural range from 2500-6000 m asl in the middle and inner Himalayas. Despite extreme inhospitable environment including low temperature and sparse vegetation, yak has successfully survived and reproduced over centuries. However, a recent decline in their population (Hedges, 2003) has raised a great concern for yak farmers and conservation scientists as the animals are of immense importance to the highland peoples of Asia, who depends on these animals for food, clothing, transportation of goods and religious causes. Although, yak over centuries, has undergone several reproductive adaptations including seasonal pattern of breeding, shorter gestation length; in general, the reproductive rate of yak is low and they are not very prolific under natural conditions of their normal habitat. Female yak attains maturity at 3 to 4 years and calves once in every two years or twice in three years, thus producing, on average, four to five calves in a lifetime. Yaks are seasonal breeders with most of the reproductive activity being restricted to the warmer part of the year (July to November). Females are seasonally polyestrous, although some cows show only a single estrous during breeding season and show estrous only in next year, irrespective of the fact whether she has calved or not. The average length of the estrous cycle is approximately 20 days with the duration of estrus less than a day. Behavioural changes in the yak cow resulting from oestrous are not usually as clear as in other domestic cattle. Gestation length is shorter than in other cattle breeds (around 258 days). The endocrinology of estrous cycle and pregnancy has been studied only recently and will be discussed in this chapter.

Male yak attains sexual maturity at an age of two to three years, although they may show mounting behaviour as early as at age of six months. Under natural condition, a bull has to establish his dominance in the mating hierarchy of the herd, before mating with a cow. Bulls reach the peak of their mating ability around the age of six to seven years. Reproductive anatomy of bull is more or less similar to that of cattle except the size of testes are smaller and testes are covered with abundant hairs. Sperm morphology and sparmatogenesis process are also similar to that of cattle. These topics have been discussed later in this chapter.

Natural service is still the predominant mating system in both wild and domestic yak. Artificial insemination has been successful in domestic yak, but its application has been restricted to some parts of China and in some organized yak farms of India. Pure breeding is fairly obligatory for yak farmers and is the main system of breeding, although crossbreeding wild yak bulls is sometime practiced by local people for breed improvement programme. Crossbreeding, at least theoretically, should be advantageous as it leads to heterosis producing hybrid vigour and negates the effect of inbreeding depression that results when pure breeding is practiced over a long time. No systematic crossbreeding, however, appears to be practised among the different breeds or local populations of yak. Recent advances in semen collection and freezing techniques has the potential to direct a more systematic breeding policy for yak. This however, needs more scientific research and extension services for practical applicability of these techniques.

Recently, a number of reproductive biotechniques, including hormonal manipulation, have been employed for augmenting reproductive efficiency of yak. Indeed, there is sufficient evidence to suggest that the reproductive rate of yak can be increased by improvements in management, feeding and assisted reproductive techniques. Towards the end of this chapter, we present glimpses of these studies which focus on the fact that this valuable animal could be well conserved and utilized for human needs with reproductive management. We still emphasize on the fact that number of such studies are less for a conclusive suggestion for increasing reproductive efficiency of yak. A generalized phenomenon of yak reproduction can only be presented after more and more such studies are being undertaken by animal scientists.

4.1. Reproductive Organs

4.1.1. Female Reproductive Organs

Female reproductive tract of yak, as like other domestic farm animals, has following parts: vestibule, vagina, cervix, uterus, oviducts and ovaries. Except for the vulva, all parts of the reproductive tract are located and suspended within the pelvic cavity with attachment from broad ligament. Broad ligament is considered the principal supporting structure and suspends the ovaries, oviducts, and uterus from either side of the dorsal wall of the pelvis. This ligament consists of mesovarium, which suspends ovaries, the mesosalpinx, which suspend oviduct and mesometrium that supports uterus within pelvic cavity. Blood vessels and nerves pass through the broad ligament to the female reproductive system. The ovarian arteries, also called utero-ovarian arteries, branch and supply blood to the ovaries, oviducts, and a portion of the uterine horns. The middle uterine artery supplies blood to rest the uterine horns and the body of the uterus. The hypogastric artery branches to supply the cervix, vagina, and vulva. The female reproductive system is supplied primarily with autonomic nerves. However, sensory nerves are found the region of the vulva, especially the clitoral region. In general, morphology and anatomy of reproductive tract of female yak have great similarity, but differs in some aspects from those of cattle. The dimensions of different reproductive organs of female yak are presented in table 4.1.

Ovary

The ovary is the primary reproductive organ of the female and serves two important reproductive functions. First is the production of the egg or ovum (oogenesis) and second is the production of estrogen and progesterone, two steroid hormones required for estrus behaviour and maintenance of pregnancy. The morphology and physiology of ovaries of female yak, to a great extent, are similar to cattle and buffaloes, although many subtle differences do exist. The ovaries of yak are oval to almond shaped organs, located in the abdominal cavity. The ovary is enclosed in a pouch like structure, the ovarian bursa. This is formed medially by mesovarium and proper ligament of ovary and laterally by utrine tube and mesosalphinx. The ovarian bursa helps to localize the ova in the neighborhood of infundibulum following ovulation. The growth of ovarian tissue is comparatively slow in yak from birth to puberty as compared to cattle. Average size and weight of ovaries of mature female are also less than cattle (Cui and Yu, 1999). The left ovary is slightly smaller than right ovary (Tian and Zhao, 2000).

Table 4.1 : Measurements of different reproductive organs of female yak

Reproductive organ	Measurement	Reference
Left ovary		
Length	2.1-2.5 cm	Tian and Zhao (2000); Cui and Yu (1999)
Weight	1.4-4.0 g	Tian and Zhao (2000) ; Cui and Yu (1999)
Right ovary		
Length	1.8-2.4 cm	Tian and Zhao (2000); Cui and Yu (1999)
Weight	1.0-4.1 g	Tian and Zhao (2000); Cui and Yu (1999)
Vagina	25-30 cm	Cai Li (1980)
Cervix		
Length	5.0±0.9 cm	Cai Li (1980)
External diameter	3.2±0.7 cm	Cai Li (1980)
Uterine tube	18 - 24 cm	Xu (1991)
Corpus uteri	2.1 ± 0.8 cm.	Cai Li (1980)

Ovarian histology of yak and cattle resembles to a great extent. Histologically, ovaries consist of layer of epithelial cells and matrix of connective tissue viz. germinal epithelium, tunica albuginea, cortex, medulla and rete ovarii. The ovary is covered by a thick tough capsule made up of the outer germinal epithelium and an inner connective tissue layer, the tunica albuginea. Germinal epithelium is mainly made up of columnar or squamous epithelial cells, which have round, oval or flat nuclei and are often rich in chromatin. Covering epithelium sometime invaginates into cortical stroma to for a tubule like structures, lined with columnar or cubical cells (Cui and Yu, 1999). Beneath the albuginea layer lays the tunica albuginea layer, which mainly consists of connective tissue. Ovarian tissue below the tunica albuginea is known as functional parenchyma. It contains ovarian follicles and the cells which produce ovarian hormones and is composed of the medulla and its outer shell, the cortex. The cortex constitutes major part of ovary and is well supplied with blood vessels. The cortex contains those cell and tissue layers associated with ovum and hormone production. Primordial follicles in yak are distributed in the peripheral part of the cortex, frequently rather close to the tunica albuginea. The medulla is composed primary of blood vessel, nerves, and connective tissue. The rete ovarii, situated in the medial part of the ovary, sometimes continues into the mesovarium. It consists of cords and ductuli, lined by epithelial cells with oval nucleus. Reti ovarii in yak has been found to be more developed in calves and heifers (Cui and Yu, 1999).

Oviduct

The oviducts are a pair of convoluted tubes extending from near the ovaries to and becoming continuous with the tips of the uterine horns. Main function of oviduct is to receive and transport egg from ovary and temporarily nourish it, until fertilization takes place. Oviduct is divided into three major parts; infundibulum, a funnel shaped structure around ovary, ampulla, the region where fertilization takes place and ishthmus, a muscular structure that joins with uterine horns. Histologically, oviduct has three main layers of tissue. The outer layer, tunica serosa, is basically composed of connective tissue. The middle layer, tunica muscularis, is composed of both circular and longitudinal smooth muscle fibers. The innermost layer, which contains both ciliated and secretory epithelial cells, is the tunica mucosa. The inner two layers have undergone specialized histological arrangement in most of the domestic livestock. This, however, has not studied in detail in yak.

Uterus

The uterus extends from utero-tubal junction to cervix. Yak has bicornuate type of uterus, characterized by a small uterine body just anterior to the cervix and two long uterine horns. The uterine body is short than that of cattle, but a long and distinct septum extends downward from the bifurcation of the uterine horn towards the uterine body (Cai Li, 1980a). Uterus has a variety of functions to perform in reproduction. Before implantation of embryo, it nourishes early stage embryo through uterine milk, secreted from endometrial glands of uterus. After implantation of embryo, placentation occurs at this site. Histologically, uterus is made up of three different layers. The outer layer, tunica serosa, is primarily constituted by connective tissue. Myometrium, the middle layer is composed of two thin longitudinal layers of smooth muscle with thicker circular layer sandwiched between them. This layer is under endocrinological control of ovary and becomes more flaccid as foetus grows. Endometrium, the inner layer has a mucosal lining along with endometrial glands. This layer and glands under influence of estrogen and progesterone undergo radical changes during estrus that causes endometrial glands to coil and branch to secrete uterine milk and preparation of the uterus for pregnancy.

Endometrium is the layer that provides functional attachment of extraembryonic membrane for supply of nutrient to the foetus as well as elimination of wastes from foetus–a mechanism called placentation. In yak, the placentation is of cotyledonary type, as in cow. The cotyledons are formed by the union of chorionic villi from the extraembryonic membranes that penetrate into caruncles, which are button-like projections on the endometrium. The placental attachment is classified as epitheliochorial means no erosion occurs either in the tissue of the extraembryonic or endometrium tissue layer during formation of the placenta. The number of cotyledons in gravid uterus of yak, however, has been found to be less as compared to that of cattle (Mohanty *et al.,* 2002).

Cervix

The cervix is a thick-walled structure that starts from body of the uterus and actually extends and protrudes back into the vagina. It contains a canal which is the opening into the uterus. Except for the period during estrus, this canal remains sealed and serves as a natural barrier for entry of microorganisms into the uterus. High levels of estrogens cause the cervical canal to dilate during estrus. Cervix is also a major sperm reservoir and thick mucus within cervical canal can filter dead and non-motile spermatozoa to reach fertilization site. The cervical canal has transverse interlocking ridges known as annular rings. The cervix of yak has few differences when compared to that of cattle. The length of cervix is slightly shorter as compared to those in cattle. The cervix has three to four transverse circles, each having many tight folds. Number of folds is higher (15-20) in outer circles than inner one (9-10). Histologically, three basic layers constitute the cervix. The outer layer of the cervix is known as tunica serosa. The middle layer is connective tissue interspersed with smooth muscle fibers. This layer gives the cervix its firm and inelastic properties. The inner mucosa layer is composed mainly of secretory epithelial cells, but some ciliated epithelial cells are present. During periparturient period, synergistic action of high levels of estrogens and relaxin causes greater dilation of cervix to ease expulsion of foetus. This dilation of the canal would appear to make the uterus more vulnerable to invading organisms. However, estrogens cause the epithelial cells of the cervix to secrete mucus that antibacterial properties, thus protecting the uterus.

Vagina

The vagina is female organ of copulation that extends from cervix to external genetalia. During natural service, semen is deposited into the anterior end of the vagina. In yak, the length of vagina is approximately 25-30 cm (Cai Li, 1980a). An elastic tubular structure, vagina has three basic layers. The outer fibrous layer, the tunica serosa, is followed by a muscular layer containing both circular and longitudinal smooth muscle fibers and an inner mucosa layer constituted by epithelial cells. These epithelial cells cornify (become cells without nuclei) under the influence of estrogens. This layer of cornified cells at the time of estrus may serve as a lubricating or protective mechanism which prevents abrasions during copulation. Under the influence of progestins, the epithelial lining regenerates.

Vulva

The vulva, or external genitalia, consists of the vestibule with related parts and the labia. The urinary duct joins the vestibule at the external urethral orifice. The labia consist of the two folds: labia minora and labia majora, female homologous for prepuce and scrotum in the male, respectively. An erectile tissue, clitoris, is located ventrally inside labia and is female homologous to the glans penis in the male. Clitoris is well supplied with sensory nerves and erects during estrus and copulation. Vestibule has vestibular glands in its posterior part that secrete lubricating mucus during copulation. The moist appearance of the vulva is due to secretions of these glands.

4.1.2 Male Reproductive Organs

The male reproductive system consists of testes, the primary reproductive organs that produce male gametes, a duct system, the secondary sex organs that carries sperm from testes to exterior and accessory glands. The testes are located in a pouch called scrotum that is suspended externally in the inguinal region. The duct system consists of duct system within testes, epididymis, vas difference, penis and urethra. The accessory gland system consists of prostate gland, seminal vesicle and Cowper's gland.

Testes

Testis, like ovary in female, serves dual function in male: production of male gamete and steroidogenesis. Development of testes originates near embryonic kidney during prenatal life. Testes, under the influence of gonadotropin and androgen, descent caudally through inguinal ring to abdomen and traverse abdominal wall to be finally placed into the scrotum. The scrotum is two-lobed sac which enclosed the testes, located in the inguinal region between the rear legs. Descent of the testes occurs because of an apparent shortening of the gubernaculum, a ligament extending from the inguinal region and attaching to the tail of the epididymis. This exterior location of testes is an adaptive evolution for maintaining proper temperature of spermatogenesis that is a few degrees less than the body temperature. Animals in which testes failed to descent (cryptorchid) are thereby sterile as spermatogenesis could not take place. Testicular artery, supplying blood to testes, form pampiniform plexus, which through a countercurrent mechanism cool off arterial blood and maintain temperature of testes below body temperature. The contraction and relaxation of dartos tunic muscle of scrotum also play a major role in maintaining scrotal temperature by dragging it in or away from body wall during cold or warmer season, respectively. The scrotum of yak has undergone further environmental adaptation to become short and hairy to maintain scrotal temperature against extreme cold climate (Qiu Zhongquan and Zhu Qimin, 1981).

Anatomical and histological structure of yak testes is similar to that of cattle, except the volume and weight of testes are lower. Average weight of yak testes is approximately 300 g (500-600 g in cattle) that is liable to change with the rate of sperm production by the organ. Histologically, testicular parenchyma is surrounded by a thick white connective tissue capsule, called tunica albuginea. Interior of testes is divided into several lobes by a tough fibrous membrane. Each lobule has highly coiled round or oblong tubules, the seminiferous tubules, embedded in the stromal tissue. The stromal tissue consists of blood vessel, nerve supply and Leydig cells, responsible for production of testosterone and small quantities of other androgens. Seminiferous tubules are the site of spermatozoa production. They contain two basic types of cells: germ cells or spermatogonia and Sertoli cells. Sertoli cells are larger and less numerous than spermatogonia. Under stimulation of FSH, Sertoli cells produce both androgen binding protein and inhibin. Their primary function is the nursing of sperm cells. Seminiferous tubules join a network of tubules, the rete testis. This tubular network is then connected to 12 to 15 small ducts, the vasa efferentia, which converge into the head of the epididymis.

Epididymis

Epididymis is the first external duct leading from the testis and extends up to vas difference. This single convoluted duct is anatomically divided into three parts: head or caput region, body or corpus region and cauda or tail region. The caput epididymidis is a flattened area at the apex of the testis, where variable number of ductules of vasa efferentia, merge into a single duct. The corpus part extends along the longitudinal axis of the testis and becomes continuous with the cauda (tail). This portion has rich secretary activity, necessary for maturation of spermatozoa, while they pass through this region. The histological structure of the epididymis is similar to that of the tubular portion of the female tract. The outer fibrous tunica serosa is followed by a smooth muscle layer, tunica muscularis. The inner most layer is epithelial layer, lined by epithelial cells. Epididymis has several roles in male reproduction. As a duct leading from the testes, the epididymis serves to transport spermatozoa. During this transportation, which takes a little longer than a week, spermatozoa undergo maturation process within epididymis. Nascent, non motile, infertile spermatozoa, after entering the caput from the vasa efferentia, gain the ability for to be both motile and fertile while they pass through the epididymis. During this process, spermatozoa lose the cytoplasmic droplet which forms on the neck of spermatozoa during spermatogenesis. The detail of maturation process has been discussed in the spermatogenesis section in this chapter. The physiological significance of the cytoplasmic droplet is not known, but it has been used as maturation indicator of spermatozoa in the epididymis. Also, concentration of spermatozoa occurs in this region through the process of fluid absorption by the epithelial cells of the epididymis. Absorption of these fluids occurs principally in the caput and proximal end of the corpus region. A third function of the epididymis is store spermatozoa in the cauda region of the epididymis. The physiological conditions viz. low pH, high viscosity, high carbon di oxide concentration, high potassium-to-sodium ratio etc. are optimum in the cauda for preserving the viability of spermatozoa for an extended period. Testosterone and probably other factors also contribute to a lower metabolic rate and extended life of spermatozoa in the cauda region.

Vas Difference and Urethra

The vas deferens is a pair of ducts leading from the distal end of the cauda of epididymis and merges with the urethra near the opening to the bladder. Near the bladder end, it has an enlarged end called ampullae, previously suggested as short term storage depot for semen. The vas deferens has a thick layer of smooth muscles in its walls and its mucosa is thrown into longitudinal folds. The ampulla region contains branched tubular glands. Vas difference is primarily associated with the function of transport of spermatozoa. It could have a possible role in fluid absorption and spermiophagy also. It seems more likely that spermatozoa may pool in the ampullae during ejaculation before being expelled into the urethra.

The urethra is common ejaculatory duct for semen and urine for male. It extends from the junction of the ampullae to the end of the penis. During ejaculation, mixing of concentrate spermatozoa from vas difference with accessory gland secretions occurs.

Accessory glands

The accessory glands viz. seminal vesicles, the prostate gland and the bulbourethral glands, are located along the pelvic portion of the urethra. Secretions of all these glands are emptied into the urethra and contribute greatly to the volume of semen. In addition, these secretions are rich in buffers, nutrients, and other substances, which contribute to the survival and optimal function of spermatozoa.

Seminal Vesicles

Seminal vesicles are compact lobulated glands that lie laterally to the terminal part of each vas differens. Fairly knobby in appearance, these glands contribute well over half of the total fluid volume of semen. Seminal vesicles are source of several unique organic compounds like fructose and sorbitol that are major sources of energy for spermatozoa. Besides, secretion from seminal vesicles is rich in phosphate and carbonate buffers that protect spermatozoa against detrimental ionic shift of semen.

Prostate Gland

The prostate is a distinct lobulated gland lying outside the thick urethral muscle, just posterior to the excretory ducts of the vesicular glands. The prostate is relatively small in the yak bull, as compared to other species, and does not produce a very large volume secretion. The secretions of the prostate are rich in inorganic ions such as sodium, chlorine, calcium, and magnesium and are responsible for maintaining osmotic balance of semen.

Bulbourethral Glands

The third accessory gland, the bulbourethral or Cowper's glands are small glands located on either side of the urethra near the point where it exits from the pelvis. In cattle, they are embedded in the bulbospongiosum muscle. The clear secretion that often drips from the penis during sexual excitement prior to service is largely produced by these glands. Secretions of bulbourethral glands contribute little to the semen volume. Their primary function is to flush and cleanse the urethra of any urine residue that may be harmful to spermatozoa.

Penis and Prepuce

The penis is the organ of copulation in males. It forms dorsally around the urethra from the point where the urethra leaves the pelvis, with the external urethral orifice at the free end of the penis. The free end of penis is called glans penis that is rich in sensory nerve supply. Yak bulls, like cattle bulls, boars, and rams have a sigmoid flexure. The sigmoid flexure is an "S" shaped anatomical structure that permits penis to be retracted completely into the body except during time of service. Strong retractor penis muscles hold the sigmoid flexure and control the effective length of penis. These retractor penis muscles arise from the vertebrae in the coccygeal region and are fused to the ventral penis just anterior to the sigmoid flexure. The penis and urethra is made up of spongy type fibroelastic erectile tissue. These cavernous (spongy) tissues are located in three regions of the penis. The corpus spongiosum penis is the cavernous tissue around the urethra. The penile bulb is covered by bulbospongiosum muscle at the base of the penis.

The corpus cavernosum penis, arising as a pair of crura from ischial arch, is a larger area of cavernous rods from the ischiocavernosus muscle. Upon sexual stimulation, arterial dilation occurs within these tissues, which cause stiffening and straightening of penis. Both the bulbospongiosum muscle and ischiocavernous muscle are striated, skeletal muscles, rather than the smooth muscle associated with most of the male and female tracts.

The prepuce is an invagination of skin which encloses the free end of the penis. It has the same embryonic origin as the labia minora in the female. It can be divided into a prepenile portion, which is the outer fold, and the penile portion, or inner folds. The orifice of the prepuce is surrounded by long and tough preputial hairs.

4.2. Reproductive Endocrinology

Endocrinology is the study of chemical communication systems that provide the means to control a huge number of physiologic processes. Like other communication networks, endocrine systems contain transmitters, signals and receivers that are called hormone producing cells, hormones and receptors, respectively. In classical term, a hormone is a physiologic, chemical substance synthesized and secreted by a ductless endocrine gland, which via circulatory system, regulates the function of a remote tissue or organ. This definition of hormone is true for most of the reproductive hormones, although organs like uterus and hypothalamus secrete hormone that do not fit into classical definition of hormone. Reproduction in mammal is greatly dependent upon coordination of nervous and endocrine systems. Unlike neural system, which mainly functions via electrical impulse, endocrine system uses chemical messengers or hormones to regulate reproduction. In this section of this chapter, we will have a brief introduction on the anatomy of endocrine glands, responsible for secretion and regulation of reproductive hormones, followed by a discussion on properties and mode of action of various reproductive hormones. Another important component of chemical signaling of reproductive processes via growth factors is not in the scope of discussion under this chapter, as these factors have not been studied in detail in yak.

4.2.1 Endocrine glands

The endocrine system comprises a series of ductless glands, each of which secretes one or several hormones that integrate body functions. The reproductive cycle of the yak is mainly coordinated by hormones produced by three primary endocrine glands: the hypothalamus, pituitary and ovary. Because of close coordination of functioning of these three glands, they have been often described as a single system –the hypothalamic-pituitary-gonadal axis (HPGA). The hypothalamic-pituitary-gonadal axis is a critical part in the regulation of reproductive processes. The hypothalamic-pituitary-gonadal pathway is regulated normally through negative feedback by hydrophobic and hydrophilic hormones.

Hypothalamus

The hypothalamus is a small cone-shaped structure located in the third ventricle region of brain, extending from optic chiasma to mammillary body. Hypothalamus is considered to be the coordinating center for most of the reproductive activities and changes. Hormones from hypothalamus have pituitary gland as their primary target organ for action. Coordination of endocrine relationship between hypothalamus and anterior pituitary is mediated by the vascular connections between these organs. A branch of the hypophyseal artery ramifies into a capillary bed in the lower hypothalamus, and hypothalmic hormones destined for the anterior pituitary are secreted into that capillary blood. Blood from those capillaries drains into hypothalamic-hypophyseal portal veins. The hypothalamic-hypophyseal portal veins branch again into another series of capillaries within the anterior pituitary. Under appropriate stimuli, hormones are released from the hypothalamus into the capillary system (hypophysial portal system) which connects the hypothalamus with the anterior pituitary.

Pituitary gland

The pituitary is located at the base of the brain in a bony depression called sella turcica. The pituitary is composed of the adenohypophysis or anterior lobe and neurohypophysis or posterior lobe. The anterior pituitary is located directly beneath the hypothalamus in a small depression of the sphenoid bone. The anterior pituitary is a classical gland composed predominantly of cells that secrete protein hormones, including the hormones related to reproduction. Anterior pituitary has five different cell types, secreting six different hormones. Among these, somatotropes secret somatotropin or growth hormone (GH), corticotropes secret adrenocorticotropic hormone (ACTH), gonado-tropes secret follicle stimulating hormone (FSH) and leutinizing hormone (LH), mammotropes secret prolactin and thyrotropes secret thyroid stimulating hormone (TSH). The posterior pituitary is not really an organ, but an extension of the hypothalamus. It is composed largely of the axons of hypothalamic neurons which extend downward as a bundle behind the anterior pituitary. It also forms the so-called pituitary stalk, which appears to suspend the anterior gland from the hypothalamus.

Gonads

The third portion of the reproductive axis consists of the gonads, testes in males and ovary in females. Gonads in both sexes, besides producing germ cells are important endocrine organs for steroidogenesis. The interstitial cells of Leydig in the seminiferous tubules of testes and theca interna cells of mature follicles are the primary cell types that produce testosterone and estrogen in male and female, respectively. After ovulation, the granulosa and theca cells are replaced by corpus luteum that secrets progesterone.

Pineal gland

Besides, endocrine glands of HPG axis, some other glands are also involved in producing hormones relevant to reproduction. Pineal gland, for example, is a gland located in roof of third ventricle of brain, which forms a solid mass located between the habenular and posterior commissures. Melatonin, the major hormone produced by the pineal gland, displays characteristic daily and seasonal patterns of secretion. These robust and predictable rhythms in circulating melatonin are strong synchronizers for the expression of numerous physiological processes in photoperiodic species. In mammals, the nighttime production of melatonin is mainly driven by the circadian clock, situated in the suprachiasmatic nucleus of the hypothalamus. The rodent superficial pineal gland is massively innervated and contains a dense network of blood vessels into which melatonin is released. However, in the deep pineal gland, being made of functional pinealocytes, melatonin could be directly released into the cerebrospinal fluid as well, as in sheep. Being made of true photoreceptors in lower vertebrates, in mammals it consists of neuroendocrine cells, the pinealocytes, with no direct light sensitivity but still expressing various photoreceptor markers (rhodopsin, S-antigen, recoverin, etc.). The mammalian pineal gland is a rather homogenous tissue containing mainly true pinealocytes (mono-, bi-, or tri-polar cells), few glial cells, phagocytic cells, and rare neurons. Melatonin is responsible for induction of cyclicity, at least in some seasonal breeders. The activity of pineal gland is influenced by dark-light cycle. The gland converts neural signal of darkness as perceived through eyes into an endocrine output of melatonin that secrets into blood and cerebrospinal fluid.

4.2.2. Reproductive Hormones

Hormones involved in reproduction can be classified into four groups, according to their biochemical composition. Protein hormones like oxytocin, FSH and LH are made up of polypeptide chains with carbohydrate residue sometime attached to them. Steroids like estrogen, testosterone are primarily derived from cholesterol. Hormones like prostaglandins are derived from fatty acids. The amine group hormones (e.g. melatonin) are derived from tyrosine or tryptophan. All the hormones coordinate via neural and endocrine feedback to regulate reproductive processes of spermatogenesis, ovulation, sexual behaviour, fertilization, implantation, gestation, parturition and lactation.

GnRH (Gonadotropin Releasing Hormone)

GnRH, also known as luteinizing hormone releasing hormone (LH-RH), is a polypeptide that is secreted from hypothalamic area. In response to neural signal, GnRH is released from the hypothalamus into the capillary system in a pulsatile manner and acts on pituitary gland for releasing FSH and LH. GnRH binds to specific receptors on gonadotrophs, and triggers the release of intracellular Ca2+, causing a transient release of both FSH and LH. GnRH controls tonic release of FSH and LH during follicular growth period as well as preovulatory surge of FSH and LH just before ovulation. Circulating concentration of estradiol has a positive feedback on release of this hormone. Elevated progesterone concentration has a negative feedback on the release of this hormone. Other factors that can alter GnRH release in the cow include temperature, photoperiod, stress and stage of the reproductive cycle (estrus, pregnancy, parturition, suckling etc.).

FSH (Follicle Stimulating Hormone)

Follicle stimulating hormone is an oligomeric glycoprotein hormone that is secreted from anterior pituitary gland. Like many other protein hormones, FSH consists of a family of related isoforms. The isoforms can be separated on the basis of size, charge, biological to immunological potency relationships, and circulatory clearance rates. FSH is an important reproductive hormone with activities including cell proliferation, inhibition of apoptosis, cellular differentiation, and stimulation of steroidogenesis. After release from the anterior pituitary, FSH travel through the animal's general circulatory system to reach the gonads. In order to activate, FSH must initially bind to its receptor within the ovary. FSH works primarily through a single G protein coupled-receptor (GPCR) although it is likely that FSH has at least three different receptors, which may be different functions. The GPCR for FSH has seven transmembrane sections, and when bound by FSH it activates adenylate cyclase through a G protein (Gs), resulting in an increase in cAMP. FSH, as the name suggest, stimulates the growth and maturation of ovarian follicles in female. FSH induces the development of several follicles until the outbreak of a dominating follicle. FSH is the key hormone stimulating the emergence of waves of follicles, and its decline is associated with selection of a dominant follicle, which then becomes dependent on LH for its final fate when concentrations of FSH are minimal. FSH induces cumulus expansion when added to bovine Cumulus oophrus complex (COCs) during in vitro maturation (IVM) and increases the developmental potential of the oocytes in terms of in vitro fertilization (IVF) outcome. The presence of FSH prevents apoptosis of bovine granulose cells in vitro, but whether this protective effect also occurs in cumulus cells is not known. FSH increases aromatase activity and consequently the biosynthesis of estradiol with in the follicle. In male, this hormone acts on germinal cells of seminiferous tubules of testes to stimulate spermatogenesis. Spermatogenesis process up to secondary spermatocyte stage is controlled by FSH. Along with LH, FSH stimulates steroid (estrogen) production from ovarian follicle. The various isoforms of FSH differ in their functional attributes. FSH is secreted from the pituitary in discrete pulses. FSH secreted in pulses is biologically more potent and alteration in concentrations of various isoforms could differently affect important reproductive functions such as the onset of puberty, stimulus for development of the preovulatory follicle etc. as the isoforms differ in their immunopotency, biopotency, receptor binding ability and circulatory clearance. Inhibins and oestradiol act directly at the anterior pituitary to decrease expression of the gene encoding the FSH subunit. Elevated level of estrogen during follicular growth has a negative feedback on tonic FSH release. This negative feedback is changed to positive with high level of estrogen just before ovulation to cause preovulatory surge of FSH and LH. Progesterone exerts a negative feedback on tonic release of FSH. Production and release of FSH can also be influenced indirectly by the same factors which can alter hypothalamic function.

Luteinizing Hormone (LH)

Luteinizing Hormone or LH is also secreted from anterior pituitary and reach gonads through systemic circulation. The hormone has some structural similarity with FSH and functions in close conjunction with FSH. The alpha subunits of LH and FSH are identical, and contain 92 amino acids. The amino acids length of beta subunits varies and this subunit is responsible for specific biologic action and interaction with the LH receptor. Tonic level of LH, with FSH stimulates secretion of estrogen by follicle in female and androgen secretion by Leydig cells of testes in male. The maintenance of Leydig cell function and androgen secretion is dependent upon pulsatile release of luteinizing hormone. Intermittent stimulation by LH is responsible for supporting differentiated function of the Leydig cell, and induction and/or maintenance of LH receptors and steroidogenic enzymes occurs with near-normal or slightly increased levels of gonadotropin. Further increases in circulating hormone levels, from either endogenous or exogenous sources, causes negative regulation of testicular LH receptors and Leydig cell responses. Theca cells in the ovary respond to LH stimulation by secretion of testosterone, which is converted into estrogen by adjacent granulosa cells. LH supports thecal cells in the ovary that provide androgens and hormonal precursors for estradiol production. However, the most important role of LH in female reproduction is the ovulation. Pulsatile release of LH is greatly enhanced just before ovulation and this 'LH surge' is responsible not only for releasing the egg, but also for initiation of the conversion of the residual follicle into a corpus luteum. LH is necessary to maintain luteal function for the first two weeks. LH is a primary factor that regulates the secretion of progesterone from corpus luteum. The action of LH at luteal cell level is mediated by its binding with specific receptor at plasma membrane level. This LH-receptor complex activates adenylate cyclase and results in elevated intracellular cAMP. An elevated level of cAMP enhances the activity of protein kinase and increased steroidogenesis. The release of LH at the pituitary gland is controlled by pulses of gonadotropin-releasing hormone (GnRH) from the hypothalamus. Those pulses, in turn, are subject to the estrogen feedback from the gonads.

Prolactin

Prolactin is a polypeptide hormone that is synthesized in and secreted from specialized cells of the anterior pituitary gland, the lactotrophs. The hormone was given its name based on the fact that an extract of bovine pituitary gland would cause growth of the crop sac and stimulate the elaboration of crop milk in pigeons or promote lactation in rabbits. Based on its genetic, structural, binding and functional properties, prolactin belongs to the prolactin/growth hormone/placental lactogen family of the helix bundle protein hormones. Prolactin is best known for the multiple effects it exerts on the mammary gland. It also affects other actions related to reproduction such as mating and maternal behaviors. The varied effects of prolactin on the mammary gland include growth and development of the mammary gland (mammogenesis), synthesis of milk (lactogenesis), and maintenance of milk secretion (galactopoiesis). It should be noted that none of these actions is solely due to prolactin, but the hormone is merely a player in an orchestra of hormones and growth factors that affect the mammary gland. In the process of lactogenesis, prolactin stimulates uptake of some amino acids, the synthesis of the milk proteins casein and á-lactalbumin, uptake of glucose, and synthesis of the milk sugar lactose as well as milk fats. In most rodents, prolactin acts as a luteotrophic hormone by maintaining the structural and functional integrity of the corpus luteum after mating. This "luteotrophic" action of prolactin, however, is not of much importance in ruminants, as LH is the primary luteotrophic hormone in these species. It has been suggested that in seasonal breeders like yak, prolactin secretion is affected by variations of day length. Circadian rhythmicity has been observed with prolactin secretion pattern in yak cows that is different from cattle and buffaloes. Whereas, in cattle and buffalo cows, higher prolactin concentrations have been recorded during day time, the diurnal prolactin pattern in yak cows indicates highest concentration around midnight and lower concentration during daytime (Prakash *et al.,* 2008). During estrous cycle, plasma prolactin concentration in yak cows although remain high at estrus; its level fluctuated throughout the cycle without any definite trend (Sarkar, 2004).

Melatonin

Melatonin, an indole amine, was first isolated from bovine pineal tissue and is secreted by the pineal gland of nearly all mammals. Melatonin in the pineal gland is synthesized from amino acid precursor tryptophan, which is converted to serotonin and then to melatonin through a series of steps. Two enzymes involved in melatonin synthesis are hydroxyindole-O-methyl-transferase and the rate limiting factor, N-acetyltransferase. Melatonin is secreted by the pineal gland with daily and seasonal rhythms mainly under the control of the circadian oscillator located in the suprachiasmatic nuclei of the hypothalamus. Secretion of this hormone is greatly enhanced at night with duration inversely proportional to the duration of the photoperiod. The target tissues and the mechanisms of action of melatonin on the reproductive axis are still not totally understood. It has been suggested that as light strikes the retina of the eye, a neural signal travels via the optic nerves to the suprachiasmatic nuclei. Optic nerves synapse with neurons of the suprachiasmatic nuclei leading to superior cervical ganglia. The daily rhythm of melatonin is considered to be a circadian mediator used by the endogenous suprachiasmatic nuclei clock to deliver the circadian message to target structures (containing melatonin receptors). Finally, melatonin secretion by the mammalian pineal gland is inhibited by the post-ganglionic neurons diverging from the superior cervical ganglia. In mammals, irrespective of their nocturnal or diurnal activity, melatonin is synthesized in the pineal gland during the dark phase of the light/dark cycle and is rapidly delivered to the body via the bloodstream. Pinealectomy does not alter the animal's circadian rhythm in rest-activity but facilitates the re-synchronization of the animal to a new photoperiod. Long daily periods of elevated secretion of melatonin has been suggested for induction of cyclicity in seasonal breeding animals. In yak cows, circadian rhythmicity in circulatory melatonin concentration has been seen with low concentration during daytime and high concentration during night during both breeding and non-breeding season (Prakash et al., 2008). Circadian rhythmicity of melatonin and prolactin secretion in yak cows has a positive correlation, although the significance of such correlation is not clearly understood (Sarkar and Prakash, 2005). Exogenous melatonin supplementation has been reported to induce cyclicity in ewes around midsummer, but this has not been demonstrated in yak.

Oxytocin

Oxytocin is a neurohypophysial hormone secreted by the hypothalamic magnocellular neurons and stored in the posterior pituitary. Oxytocin is synthesized as part of a prohormone (oxytocin-neurophysin I) that is packaged into neurosecretory granules and transported via axons to the posterior pituitary gland. Oxytocin and its carrier molecule are stored in axon terminals located in the posterior pituitary until their release into the blood stream. Oxytocin has been traditionally recognized as a 'female' hormone involved in milk ejection, parturition and induction of luteolysis in conjunction with prostaglandin (F2á). The primary role of oxytocin is to reflex release of milk (milk let down). Upon tactile and visual stimuli associated with suckling, oxytocin releases in to the blood and causes contraction of myoepithelial cells to release milk. Oxytocin is a potent endogenous uterine stimulating hormone and pregnant uterus is an important target organ for it. Action of oxytocin may be direct, through the activation of myosin light chain kinase or indirect by stimulating the synthesis of prostaglandin F2á. In the bovine, myometrial oxytocin receptor increase substantially as early as mid-gestation, but show no marked increase thereafter until parturition. Endometrial oxytocin receptor concentrations, however, increase markedly near term of pregnancy. Plasma levels of oxytocin in parturient cows have been found to increase sharply near the time of expulsion of the calf suggesting its role in the final stages of parturition.

Oxytocin has been found to be synthesized by the corpus luteum of a number of mammalian species including ruminants. Although luteal oxytocin may indirectly promote luteolysis to establish the normal estrous cycle, in-vitro studies have shown that oxytocin, in a dose-dependent manner, significantly increased progesterone production by cultured granulosa cells of bovine preovulatory follicles.

Oxytocin has several important functions in male reproduction, including sexual behaviour and transportation of sperm. Oxytocin is a potent agent known to induce penile erection. In several animals including the human, a pulse of oxytocin, probably of hypothalamic origin is associated with ejaculation. Oxytocin has been postulated to modulate contractility of the male tract to regulate sperm transport and maturation within seminiferous tubules and epididymis. Spermatozoa are immotile within the male tract and hence need to be transported from the testis following spermiation. Oxytocin enhances both type A (high frequency movements like ripples of the tubule walls) and type B (large contractions associated with bulk movements of the seminal contents) movements of seminiferous tubules. Oxytocin increases cauda epididymal contractility in vitro suggesting that it may have a role in the propulsion of sperm from the cauda to the vas deferens at ejaculation. Oxytocin has been shown to modulate mitotic activity in various organs including bone osteoblasts, mammary glands and ovary.

Gonadal Hormones

Gonads, testes and ovaries, primarily secret steroidal hormones with some protein hormones (inhibin and relaxin). Steroid hormones are primarily secreted by gonads, with placenta and adrenal cortex secreting these hormones to some extent. There are three basic types of steroids viz. androgens, estrogens and progestins, all having a common cyclopentanoperhydrophenanthrene nucleus in their chemical structure. These hormones have a common biosynthetic pathway with 18 carbon steroids showing estrogenic activity, 19 carbon steroids showing androgenic activity and 21 carbon steroids showing progestogen properties. The secretary activity of gonadal steroids is under endocrine control of anterior pituitary.

Estrogens

Estrogens are a group of steroid hormones that derived names because of their close association with estrus. The three major naturally occurring estrogens are estradiol-â, estrone, and estriol, with estradiol being the predominate and biologically active form in females. Estrogens are produced primarily by developing follicles in the ovaries, the corpus luteum, and the placenta. Estrogens have long been considered to be specific female hormones; however, the presence of estrogens in the male gonad has been well documented. Synthesis of estrogens starts in theca interna cells in the ovary through a common biosynthetic pathway for all gonadal hormones. In this pathway, androstenedione is produced from cholesterol that crosses the basal membrane into the surrounding granulosa cells and is converted to estrone or estradiol, either immediately or through testosterone. The conversion of testosterone to estradiol, and of androstenedione to estrone, is catalyzed by the enzyme aromatase. This microsomal enzymatic complex is composed of a specific heme-glycoprotein (P450arom) that functions with a ubiquitous reductase as an electron donor. Like all steroid hormones, estrogens readily diffuse across the cell membrane. Once inside the cell, they bind to and activate estrogen receptors. Estrogens act via two types of receptors, ER-α and ER-β. The ovary contains both ER subtypes, with a predominance of ER-β over ER-α in granulosa cells. Testicular cells also contain both types of receptor with the predominance of ER-β in the testicular cells, particularly gonocytes, pachytene spermatocytes, and spermatids.

Estrogen is the primary female reproductive hormone that performs a variety of reproductive functions. In general, it stimulates development of secondary sex characteristics, mammary gland development along with progesterone, uterine development, maturation of fallopian tubes, maturation of the skeleton and increased fat deposition. In the absence of estrogen, the female-specific phenotype of the ovarian cells is lost and a more testicular type of appearance is noted. Estrogen has acknowledged local intrafollicular actions. It has direct proliferative and differentiative influences on follicle development, depending on the stage of folliculogenesis. From the experiment on ER-α and ER-β knockout mice it has been suggested that the proliferative actions of estradiol require ER-α, whereas the differentiative (and antiproliferative) effects of estradiol are mediated principally by ER-β. The actions of estrogen are intimately related to the actions of follicle-stimulating hormone (FSH) in folliculogenesis. The specific genes induced in granulosa cells by estradiol have not been identified, but it is clear that estradiol exerts a supporting role on FSH action.

The widespread distribution of estrogen receptors in testicular cells indicates a possible estrogen regulation of male reproductive functions. Recently, estradiol involvement has been explored in several steps of sperm production and maturation. To exert their effects, testicular or locally produced estrogens interact with specific estrogen receptors, which in turn modulate the transcription of specific genes involved in cell growth, function, and differentiation. In vitro studies have shown that the multiplication of rat gonocytes is in part regulated by estradiol. Estrogens also seem necessary for the achievement of fertility of the male rodent. Estrogens, through the modulation of aquaporin-1 expression, are involved in the regulation of fluid reabsorption in the proximal regions of the rat and monkey epididymides. The lack of fluid reabsorption leads to an accumulation of fluid within seminiferous tubules and therefore induces an increase in pressure that can in turn destroy germ cells. In ram, the estradiol concentration in the testicular vein is positively correlated with the daily production of primary spermatocytes per testis.

Progesterone

Progesterone is the gonadal hormone secreted principally by corpus luteum. Progesterone is major member of progestin group of hormones, which converts the estrogen-primed endometrium to establish and maintain pregnancy in animals after fertilization. Progesterone is synthesized through common biosynthetic pathway for other gonadal steroids. Progestin nucleus may be synthesized from simple carbon compounds. The intermediate compounds probably include acetoacetate, hydroxymethylglutarate, and squalene, which is a precursor of the cholestane series of compounds. Cholesterol is probably hydroxylated at the C-20 position and cleaved at the 21 carbon by a bovine side-chain desmolase. The resulting pregnenolone is converted by two enzymes to progesterone. For many years progesterone (?4-pregnene - 3, 20-dione) was thought to be the only naturally occurring progestational agent. In recent years, however, several other compounds have been isolated. The most important of these are 20 α-hydroxy- ?4- pregnene-3-one (20 α-ol), 20 β-hydroxy-?4-pregnene-3-oue (20 β-ol) and 17 α-hydroxy- ?4- pregnene-3, 20-dione (17-hydroxyprogesterone). After release into the blood stream, progesterone is weakly but mostly bound to plasma proteins that accounts for most of the circulating progesterone. Of the remainder, progesterone is strongly bound to transcortin. Physiological effects of progesterone are mediated by interaction of the hormone with specific intracellular progesterone receptors (PRs) that are expressed as two protein isoforms, PR-A and PR-B. Both proteins arise from the same gene and are members of the nuclear receptor superfamily of transcription factors.

Progesterone regulates several important reproductive functions such as maintenance of pregnancy, induction of ovulatory heat, development of mammary glands, suppression of uterine motility etc. The most dramatic role of progesterone probably occurs during pregnancy. As the name of the steroid implies, it favors gestation, at least in early pregnancy in all species. Progesterone is essential for the uterine development necessary for implantation, blastocyst development, and maintenance of the fetus and of uterine tone during pregnancy. Progesterone acts on the endometrium, inhibiting myometrial activity and causing preparation for implantation regardless of whether or not a zygote is present. Progesterone has been suggested for decades as a mediator of the ovulatory response. This is probably indirect through its effect on LH release. Inhibitors of enzymes necessary for progesterone synthesis, P450 side chain cleavage (P450scc) and 3β-hydroxysteroid dehydrogenase (3β-HSD) inhibit ovulation and the block can be overcome with exogenous progesterone. Progesterone probably has an effect on tubal and uterine transport of sperm and ova. Mating behavior is most effectively precipitated by a combination of estrogen and progesterone in various animal species. Progesterone appears to increase the quantity and quality of nest building and the retrieval of offspring in rats and mice. Progesterone favors an economy of body metabolism increases the efficiency of nutrient utilization especially during pregnancy.

Androgens

Androgen is the generic term for steroid derivatives of androstane (19-carbon tetracyclic hydrocarbon nucleus) responsible for development and maintenance of masculine characteristics in vertebrates. The primary androgen is testosterone, synthesized by Leydig cells of testes, besides dehydroepiandrosterone (DHEA), dehydroepiandrosterone sulfate (DHEA-S), and androstenedione, which are synthesized by the adrenal cortex. Leydig cells produce bulk of testicular testosterone from cholesterol precursor with enzymes that are sequestered in Leydig cell mitochondria and smooth endoplasmic reticulum. Androgens, primarily androstenedione and testosterone, are also produced by theca cells in response to LH. Testosterone, although primary, is not biologically active form. Dihydrotestosterone (DHT), a metabolite of testosterone, is actually a more potent androgen and binds more strongly to androgen receptors. Testosterone in blood, either circulates free, loosely bound to albumin or tightly bound to androgen-binding protein (ABP). ABP is a testicular glycoprotein that binds androgens with high affinity and transports them to the epididymis. Free testosterone is converted to dihydrotestosterone (DHT) via 5á-reductase before binding to nuclear androgen receptors (AR). The AR functions only after binding its hormonal ligands (androgens), which induce transformation of the receptor and results in dimerization, nuclear localization and DNA binding.

Testosterone, as a primary gonadal steroid in male, controls several vital reproductive processes including stimulation of spermatogenesis and prolonging lifespan of epididymal spermatozoa. In addition to playing a key role in testis descent, androgens are responsible for the stabilization and differentiation of the Wolffian ducts (the internal reproductive system) and for regulating the differentiation of external genitalia and the prostate. Androgens have been shown to have a stimulatory effect on Sertoli cell proliferation. It promotes growth, development and secretory activities of accessory sex organs in male. This hormone is responsible for libido and penile erection in males. The anabolic actions of androgens can enhance muscle strength and increase muscle size. The AR is present in skeletal muscle and, more specifically, has been found in satellite cells. During development and regeneration, quiescent satellite cells are activated and start proliferating under influence of androgens, at which stage they are often referred to as myogenic precursor cells or myoblasts, which further differentiate into post-mitotic myotubes that eventually fuse with myofibers.

Besides obligatory role as an estrogen precursor, androgens in females are directly involved in female reproductive physiology. In the early stages of folliculogenesis, androgens appear to promote follicular growth. Testosterone has a role in follicular recruitment by decreasing the numbers of primordial follicles and enhancing the numbers of follicles at other stages of development. Apart from effects on growth, androgens have been shown to enhance the follicle stimulating hormone (FSH)-mediated differentiation of granulosa cells, as indicated by an increase in progesterone and oestradiol production and to play roles in oocyte maturation. Testosterone and dihydrotestosterone (DHT) have an effect on ovulation rate. DHT acts through the androgen receptor to increase FSH receptors and FSH secretion, which could both help in the maturation process of follicles.

Inhibins

Inhibin is a heterodimeric glycoprotein that was originally characterized as suppressing follicle-stimulating hormone (FSH) secretion. Inhibins, like other members of the transforming growth factor β (TGF-β) superfamily, are disulphide-linked dimer of an alpha subunit and a beta subunit. The inhibin family is further complicated by the existence of two isoforms of β-subunit, β A subunit and the β B subunit. Thus there are two 'types' of inhibin, inhibin-A or inhibin-B. To date, the inhibin-B forms have been detected and measured in humans and other primates, but have not yet been detected in ruminants. While inhibins are dimers of alpha and beta subunits, dimers of beta-beta subunits form activin, another hormone with antagonizing effect against inhibin. Activin is a general growth-stimulating factor, and additionally, activin stimulates FSH secretion, thus antagonizing the main biological action of inhibin. Inhibin is produced by the Sertoli cells of the testis and granulose cells of the ovary in response to FSH. In accordance with the negative feedback relationship between inhibin and FSH, inhibin secretion is increased by FSH. Other factors have been shown to influence inhibin secretion. Estradiol stimulates inhibin- A but not inhibin-B in rats, and IGF-1 increases alpha subunit expression. The hormone is found in blood plasma, although difficult to detect, and in great quantities in seminal plasma and follicular fluid. Not all of the circulating inhibin is in the biologically active (dimeric) form. In ruminants, there is a vast amount of 'free' alpha subunit in the blood and follicular fluid. This free alpha subunit has no known biological action. Recent research has suggested that inhibin operates by two mechanisms. It actively compete with activin for activin receptors (both having a common β-subunit), which results in an antagonistic action. The second is by interaction with specific and high affinity receptors, which activate signal transducing pathways that oppose activin action. Additional inhibin-binding proteins may be involved in either process.

Inhibin performs several important reproductive functions in ruminants. Originally identified as gonadal factor that influence the production of follicle-stimulating hormone in the pituitary, subsequently, inhibin has been shown to play complex roles in neuroendocrine regulation and also modulate luteotropic hormone, growth hormone and adrenocorticotropic hormone production. Inhibin negatively regulates secretion of FSH to a level, optimum for maintaining species specific number of ovulations in both single and litter bearing species. In addition, it affects gonadal functions such as steroid production and regulates placental hormone synthesis. In these processes, inhibin has a common and generally antagonistic interaction with activin. Studies in mice have shown that inactivation of the activin/inhibin β B gene results in incomplete mammary development as evident through incomplete ductal elongation and morphogenesis of secretory alveoli and consequently failure of lactation (Robinson and Hennighausen, 1997). As inhibin acts systemically to inhibit FSH release, it has been postulated that a reduction of inhibin secretion would increase FSH concentrations and thus offer potential for multiple ovulations and fecundity percentage of animals. Domestic ruminants have been immunized against a variety of inhibin preparations, and small increases in ovulation rate have been reported in cattle, sheep and goats.

4.3. Reproductive Processes

4.3.1. Puberty

In a broad sense puberty is a multifactorial process of physical maturation resulting in reproductive readiness. Puberty is achieved when sexual maturation has progressed to the point where insemination and fertilization can be accomplished. In terms of endocrine profile, long before puberty, pituitary can respond to GnRH, but the frequency of GnRH release from hypothalamus is low mainly due to negative feedback by gonadal steroids. As the animal approaches puberty, negative feedback of steroids on secretion of gonadotropins by the pituitary declines and this permits an increase in the frequency of gonadotropins pulses from hypothalamus. It has been suggested that this negative blockade of HPG axis is removed during puberty as number of steroid receptors, through which steroids exerts it's negative feed back decrease in hypothalamus, while sensitivity of pituitary gland to GnRH increases. This results in increased frequency of gonadotropins pulses and beginning of cyclic activity in animals.

Puberty in bulls has been defined as the phase of bodily development during which the gonads secrete hormones in amounts sufficient to cause accelerated growth of the genital organs and the appearance of secondary sexual characters. The accepted definition for onset of puberty in bovine bulls has been further refined to include the age at which they first produce an ejaculate containing at least 50 million sperm, having a minimum of 10 percent individual progressive motility (Wolf *et al.,* 1965). Yak males start to show mounting behaviour around the age of six months, and this behaviour intensifies in the following year, although no sperm have been found in the epididymal fluid of yak bulls before the age of two years. Thus, in real sense bulls are considered to reach puberty around the age of 2½ - 3 years when bulls are capable of a successful mating. This normally occurs in the third and fourth breeding season, and bulls reach their peak ability at around six to seven years old. Studies in yaks suggest that spermatogonia begin to differentiate at 12 months of age and that sperm are present in the epididymis by 18 months of age. However, the LDH-x band, a marker characteristic of sexual maturity in mammals, is not present until 24 months of age. The age at which a yak bull is able to mate is dependent on several factors including breed, nutritional status and herd size. Under natural conditions, a male is not able to mate with a female until it establish its dominant position in the in the mating hierarchy by fighting with herd mates. It has been found that Maiwa yak bulls could be used for mating from three years old onward (Cai Bolin, 1981), whereas, Zhongdian yak bulls could be used for mating when they are four years old (Zhonxuan and Fenying, 1982). Study showed that the ejaculate volume and the concentration and motility of sperm in the semen rise steadily from the age of three to nine years and then declined (Yun, 1994). Mating frequencies of younger bulls (3-5 years of age) have been reported to be higher than older bulls. Therefore, it is apparent that younger bulls have a comparable fertilizing ability as the older bulls because fertilization seemed to be more dependent on the number of services than on the age of the bull, in line with the pregnancy results (Magesh, 1990).

In females, puberty is defined as the time when the heifer has her first ovulation. First estrus in yak females generally occurs in the second to the fourth-warm season following birth, at ages between 13 and 36 months in yak production areas (Katiyar and Sinha, 1983; Zhang *et al.*, 1997; Sarbagishev *et al.*, 1989). Puberty as evident through onset of first oestrous is determined more by body development at the beginning of the breeding season than by age. It has been found that females of same breed could have a different pubertal age and fast growing animal that attains 60-80 percent of mature weight enter puberty at an age of 2-3 years, whereas slowing growing animals start cyclic activity at an age of 48-54 months (Zi *et al.*, 1996). In China, the majority of yaks are mated for the first time at the age of three years – in the fourth warm season following birth, but under favourable conditions some yak may be mated a year earlier. First mating at the age of two years, though it also occurs in China, is more common among yak in some other countries like Bhutan, Buryatia etc.

It is apparent that age of puberty in yak is a complex interaction of breed, nutritional status and other environmental factors. Season of birth also has a significant effect on the age at which puberty occurs. Evidence indicates that calves born from March to the beginning of May can have their first cycle in the breeding season of the following year (i.e. at 15 or 16 months of age), while those born late in the season may not have their first estrus until 25 or 26 months of age (Katzina and Maturova, 1989). Nutritional supplementation during winter can significantly increase growth rate and hence advance puberty (Cheng and Liu, 1994). The variation in timing of puberty among different breeds is likely to result from their different genetic backgrounds.

Table 4.2 : Semen characteristics of yak

Colour	Volume	Sperm concentration	pH	Progressive Motility (%)	Abnormal Sperm (%)	Total N content	Viscosity	Reference
Milky-white	2 - 5 ml	7.5-16.0 × 10^8/ml	6.4 - 6.7	70 – 85	5.1 - 10.0	1334 mg/100ml	1.17 centipoise	Zhang (2000)
-	2.4 ± 0.9 ml	2680 ± 590 × 10^6/ml	-	82± 5.0	6.3 -10.4	-	-	Du Fusheng (1987)
Milky white	3-4.5 ml	150-220×10^6/ml	6.3-6.6	70-86	10-25	-	-	Das and Sarkar (2004)
Milky-white to slightly yellow	-	2.13x10^{10}/ml	6.6	63	6.3	1437.7mg/100ml	1.169 centipoise	Lu (2000)*
-	2.7 ± 0.3 ml	968 ± 233 × 10^6/ml		82.3 ± 0.9				Sarkar *et al.*, (2009)

* Wild yak semen

4.3.2. Sperm and Semen

Sperm Morphology

Spermatozoa are a specifically differentiated cell with remarkable structural features and carrying unique molecules enabling them to fertilize an ovum. Typical structure of a sperm has three segments: head, neck and tail. The sperm head contains the nucleus, the acrosome, a small amount of the cytoplasm and the cytoskeleton. The nucleus carries the paternal genetic information in form of highly condensed DNA bound to with arginine and cysteine-rich protein called protamines. The disulfide bonds between the sperm DNA and the basic cysteine residues of the protamines enable the compaction and the stability of the sperm DNA. As a result, the sperm DNA is stable and completely inactive and does not replicate until after the sperm enters the egg. The acrosome, a unique structure of the sperm head originating from the Golgi apparatus, covers the anterior portion of the nucleus and contains a variety of hydrolytic enzymes and proteases. Following the release of these enzymes after acrosome reaction, spermatozoa penetrate the zona pellucida surrounding the oocyte. In yaks, the head of a sperm has a reverse oval shape. The front two-thirds are enclosed by the acrosome, the nucleus is located in the middle and the final one-third lies in the post nuclear cap (Yan, 2000). The membrane of the acrosome can be regionally divided into the outer acrosomal membrane (OAM), lying directly underneath the plasma membrane and the inner acrosomal membrane (IAM), overlying the nuclear envelop. The postacrosomal sheath covers the region of the sperm head below the equator (Xia, 1990). During the acrosome reaction, the OAM and the apical plasma membrane, above the equatorial segment, fuse at multiple sites and create openings on the membrane, through which the acrosomal contents are released. The dimensions of head of yak sperm have been reported to be 7.74 - 8.10 μm in length and 4.1 μm thick at its widest point (Zhu *et al.,* 1988). The neck is the connecting segment between head and tail of sperm and is formed as depression of middle of the lower part of the sperm's head. It consists of nine outer-segment, cylinder-shaped implantation plates. The sperm tail may be divided into three distinct regions—the midpiece, characterized by the highly packed helical array of mitochondria surrounding the central cytoskeletal framework of the tail; the principal piece distal to the midpiece; the end piece, the shortest and the most distal part of the tail. The full length of the tail contains a central axial filament called the axoneme. The axial filament consists of 9 thick fibrils, 9 microtubule doublets and 2 center microtubules. The other important cytoskeletal features of the sperm tail are the outer dense fibers, the mitochondrial sheath, and the fibrous sheath. The mitochondrial sheath is comprised of a mitochondrial helix covered by a protoplasmic membrane. The principal piece is made up by the mid-axial filament and fibrils sheath. The telopiece of sperm has lost the fibrils sheath and the thick fiber; the only structure remaining is the mid axial-filament covered by a protoplasmic membrane. When compared to morphology of Taurus cattle sperm, the midpiece of yak sperm has slightly shorter length, whereas, its principle piece has greater length than cattle sperm (Xia, 1990). The tail is the propeller of sperm tail that facilitates the locomotion. This motility is an indispensable component of sperm's fertilization capacity.

Spermatogenesis

Spermatozoa develop in the seminiferous tubules of the testis through a series of precise cell division and differentiation process called spermatogenesis. The whole process of spermatogenesis can be divided into three distinctive phases:

(i) *Spermatocytogenesis*: involves cellular division including the proliferation and meiotic division of stem cell, spermatogonia, resulting into formation of haploid spermatids.

(ii) *Spermiogenesis*: involve the metamorphic process by which spermatids undergo structural and developmental changes to form spermatozoa.

(iii) *Spermiation*: the process of release of formed spermatozoa into the lumen of seminiferous tubules.

Spermatocytogenesis

The seminiferous tubules, site of spertocytogenesis, contain two types of cells: the small, rounded spermatogonia, which are the potential gametes and larger somatic Sertoli cells, which play a supporting role during both spermatocytogenesis and spermiogenesis. Xia (1990a) concluded that the numbers of both Sertoli cells and all kinds of germ cells in yak testes are approximately 80 percent of those in cattle. After migrating to the embryonic testes, primordial germ cells will undergo a number of mitotic divisions before forming gonocytes. At puberty gonocytes will differentiate into A0 spermatogonia, which progressively divide to give rise A1 and A2 type spermatogonia. The A2 spermatoginium will divide, forming a dormant (A1) and an active (A3) spermatogonium and starting a new generation of developing germ cells. The active spermatogonium will undergo four mitotic divisions eventually forming 16 primary spermatocytes. On entering meiosis, the primary diploid spermatocyte replicates its DNA content. The long prophase is usually divided into different stages. They are, in chronological order, preleptotene (DNA replication), leptotene (condensation of chromosome), zygotene (pairing up of homologous chromosomes), pachytene (combination of maternal and paternal homologous chromosomes), diplotene (desynapsis). After the diplotene stage the two meiotic divisions rapidly occur, leading to four haploid round spermatids. Thus, four spermatids form from each primary spermatocyte, or 64 from each active (A3) spermatogonium. Since A1 spermatogonia divide by mitosis to from A2 spermatogonia, the potential yield of spermatids is higher than is actually realized. Degeneration of spermatogonia during mitotic divisions accounts for this loss in efficiency. In yak, the average production rate of round spermatids has been reported to be 26.95 (42.1% of the theoretical yield) from a single spermatogonium A (Xia, 1990a). The numbers of primary spermatocytes remain relatively stable at the stage of proleptonema, leptonema, zygotene, and the long pachytene period. On average, 30.8 secondary spermatocytes in each seminiferous tubule cross section have been reported in yaks, close to double the number of primary spermatocytes. This indicates that few cells at this stage are lost by degeneration. However, these form 55.4 spermatids, indicating that losses during meiosis are approximately 10 percent of the theoretical value (Xia, 1990a; Liu, 1993).

Spermiogenesis

Spermiogenesis is the process by which the haploid round spermatids undergo dramatic structural changes including the formation of the acrosome, axonemal assembly, nuclear elongation, chromatin condensation, the assembly of other accessory components such as the mitochondria around the axoneme and reduction of cytoplasmic volume to become the highly-specialized, hydrodynamic, mature spermatozoa. Events associated with this process can be divided into four phases: golgi phase, cap phase, acrosomal phase and maturation phase. The golgi phase is characterized by formation of acrosomal granules and coalescence of granules into a single acrosomal granule. Acrosomal granule is subsequently enclosed by a nuclear envelope. Early stage of tail formation starts in this phase.

Cap phase is characterized by spreading of acrosomal granule over the surface of spermatid nucleus until it covers two thirds of anterior portion of spermatid nucleus. Axonemal components of tail start forming in this phase. Acrosomal phase is associated with some major developmental processes that include genesis of acrosomal sac, tail formation, nuclear elongation, organization of mitochondria around the axoneme to form mitochondrial sheath. Cytoplasm is displaced to caudal aspect of nucleus where it surrounds the proximal part of developing tail. Finally, the maturation phase involves transformation of the elongated spermatids into spermatozoa to be released into the lumen of seminiferous tubule. The chromatin materials undergo condensation to form sperm nucleus and a fibrous sheath is formed around axoneme. The mitochondria become tightly packed into a continuous mitochondrial sheath. After this stage spermatozoa are ready to be released into the lumen of seminiferous tubules.

Spermiation

Spermiation is the process by which the newly formed spermatozoa are released into the lumen of the seminiferous tubules by spermiation. The elongated spermatids are gradually extruded into the lumen of seminiferous tubules. The cytoplasm eventually forms a cytoplasmic droplet in the neck region of released spermatozoa. Following release of spermatozoa, the residual bodies are phagocytized by Sartoli cells for recycling of protoplasmic components. The successful completion of spermatogenesis requires a unique environment within the seminiferous tubule. This is achieved through the organization of Sertoli cells, which forms the blood-testis barrier by the tight junction formed between adjacent Sertoli cells. The Sertoli cells provide spermatogonia the necessary nutritional, physical, and hormonal supplies to undergo spermatogenesis.

A number of hormones including FSH, LH and testosterone play important role in spermatogenesis. The roles of these hormones have been discussed in the reproductive hormone section. In general, LH plays an indirect role in spermatogenesis through stimulation of the release of testosterone from cells of Leydig. Testosterone and FSH then act on the seminiferous tubules to stimulate spermatogenesis. FSH appears more dominant in regulating spermiogenesis. Both testosterone and FSH may exert their influence directly through germ cells and/or indirectly through Sertoli cells. FSH stimulates the Sertoli cells to secrete both androgen binding protein (ABP) and inhibin. Feedback control operates on HPG axis in regulating the spermatogenesis process. Testosterone has a negative feedback effect on the hypothalamus and anterior pituitary. High concentrations of testosterone will inhibit the release of GnRH, FSH, and LH, whereas low concentrations permit their release. It has been demonstrated that PGF2αwill stimulate the release of LH and testosterone. Therefore, PGF2α may be involved in the feedback regulation between the hypothalamus, anterior pituitary, and testes.

Spermatogenic Cycle

Spermatozoa are being continuously formed and released into the duct system. Therefore, at any given time, spermatozoa at different stage of development will be found in a transverse section of seminiferous tubule. These are arranged concentrically with layers of spermatogonia near the wall of seminiferous tubules followed by spermatocytes and spermatids in layers progressing toward the lumen. It has been observed that a kind of synchrony exists in organization of different kind of spermatozoa and certain stages are always associated. Because these cell types are always associated together and reappear in series with cyclic regularity through a cross section of the seminiferous tubules, they can be classified. One such classification, the spermatogenetic cycle includes 12 different stages of cellular associations that occur between two appearances of the same developmental stage. Xia (1990b) reported that the spermatogenetic cycle of yak bulls are very similar to that in cattle. It appears that the VII phase and the XI phase are very long, yet the IX, X, and XII phase are rather shorter. The organization of germ cells in the seminiferous tubules through space and over time are important to the continuity of sperm production.

Semen Quality

The specialized sperm cells, after a complex differentiation process, mix with secretions from accessory glands and come out as semen during ejaculation. The liquid suspension which is formed during ejaculation is called seminal plasma. The quality of semen depends upon a number of genetic and environmental factors and is extremely important for successful fertilization process. The colour of yak semen varies from milky white to light yellow. Average volume of semen is 2-2.5 ml, when collected by artificial vagina method, much lower that obtained by a standard collection from a cattle bull (5-8 ml). So far, Electro-ejaculation method is not much effective for yak and yield only some amount of fluid was obtained with very few to nil spermatozoa. The quality of semen varies from breed to breed, age and seasonal changes. It has been observed that best quality semen is produced during autumn than other parts of the year. This improved quality is associated with plasma testosterone level of bulls (Sarkar *et al.,* 2009). The characteristic of yak semen, as studied by different researchers, is presented in table 4.3.

Table 4.3 : Duration of Estrous cycle and associated events in yak

Length of estrous cycle (day)	Duration of estrus	Ovulation time (after end of estrus)	Reference
19.1 (10 - 28)	3.7 days (1 to 6 days)	-	Katzina and Maturova, (1989)
20.0 ± 4.0	0.5-18.5 h	-	Purevzav and Beshlebnov, (1967)
20-22	9-23 h	28-34 h	Sarkar and Prakash (2005); Sarkar et al. (2006)
19-21	12-36 h	12-36 h	Yu et al. (1993)
7-29	16-48 h	-	Yu (1983)
20-28	1-3 days	-	Cai Li (1981)
20.1 ± 8.2	1.9 ± 1 day	-	Liu and Liu, (1982)

4.3.3. Follicular development

The follicle is the ovarian part that enables ovary to perform its dual function of gametogenesis and steroidogenesis. Follicles form in the ovary when developmentally arrested germ cells or oocytes recruit somatic follicular cells and organize into discrete 'resting' primordial follicles. These follicles evolve through a complex series of proliferative and differentiative steps called folliculogenesis, to a structure and state where ovulation is feasible, or they succumb to atresia and die. Typical structure of follicle comprises of an oocyte surrounded by a varied number of layers of granulose cells, an antrum formed during growth of follicle and liquor folliculi, fluid that fills the antrum. Follicular fluids play a major role in initiation of follicular growth, steroidogenesis and nuclear and cytoplasmic maturation of oocyte. As the follicle grows, the connective tissue around follicle forms theca layer that later differentiates into theca externa and theca interna. Most of the follicular reserve of mammals undergoes atresia and a few could lead to become fully matured Graafian follicle that during ovulation releases the ovum. A follicle has to pass several stages of maturation before it becomes a "ripped" follicle to release oocyte during ovulation.

The ovary of yak, like cattle contains primodial, secondary or growing and Graafian follicles. The primodial follicles, the predominant type of follicle in foetus and neonates, differentiate from primordial germ cells (oogonia). Oocyte within primodial follicle is centrally located and remains in an arrested stage of cell division (first meiotic prophase). Primordial follicles in yak are distributed in the peripheral part of the cortex, often close to the tunica albuginea. Primordial follicles usually contain one, but occasionally two oocytes surrounded by a single layer of squamous epithelial cells. In newborn calves, primordial follicles are generally distributed in groups called egg nests, each group having a cluster of 10 or more follicles (Cui and Yu, 1999). The diameter of primodial follicle in newborn yak calves ranges between 25-30 ìm. Average reserves of primodial follicles in one month old calves is around 53500 which drastically deplete to become less than half at age of maturity (Cui and Yu, 1999). Secondary or growing follicles are characterized by two or more layers of granulosa cells. After formation of three or four layers of granulose cells around oocyte, the cylindrical granulosa cells of basement membrane start to arrange orientally. A layer of spindle like squamous fibrous cells which surround the granulosa cells from outside start developing into early theca interna layer (Cui and Yu, 1999). Fluid formation around the oocyte and granulosa cell layers begins at this stage. Follicle size at this stage ranges between 145 - 180ìm. Further growth of growing follicle leads to the formation of young Graafian follicle, which is characterized by an antrum. The antrum is a space among the follicular cells, which appears when follicles reach about 0.2 mm in diameter. The antrum is filled with a fluid, the liquor folliculi, and gradually increases in size by the accumulation of fluid. Follicular fluid is rich in steroids and glycoproteins, secreted by cells of follicular wall and serves several important functions. It regulates function of granulosa cells and initiates steroidogenesis. It helps in oocyte maturation, ovulation and prepare the follicle for formation of corpus luteum after ovulation takes place. In yak, complete antrum formation occurs when the follicle reaches size of about 300-500 ìm. The granulosa cell layer close to basement membrane has larger granulosa cells than other layers with regularly arranged nuclei that form a "dotted line" around the granulosa cell layers. The oocyte within the follicle rests on a cluster of granulosa cells that form cumulus oophorus. The granulosa cell layers, from outside, are covered by theca layers. Theca layers have two parts: theca interna and theca externa, with almost indistinct boundaries between them.

As the follicle grows, the oocyte within it undergoes several stages of development to prepare itself for fertilization process. This process of maturation of oocyte, as it called, involves two stages: a period of growth and a period of nuclear and cytoplasmic maturation. At birth, the cell division of oocyte remains arrested at first meiotic prophase stage. Oocyte at this stage is immature, incapable of fertilization and is called primary oocyte. After puberty, when cyclicity begins in a mature female, upon selection and recruitment of a primordial follicle for further growth, the oocyte and its follicle begin to grow. This cytomorphologic growth of oocyte involves increase of its size, formation of external membrane (zona pellucida) with close cooperation from cumulus cells. The nuclear division, however, still remained suspended in diplotene stage of first meiotic prophase until gonadotropin ovulatory surge occurs. The meiotic inhibiting effect of granulosa cells on oocyte is suppressed by ovulatory surge of gonadotropin, which involves metabolic modification of follicular layer. Meiosis progresses from first meiotic prophase to metaphase of second meiotic division, where it suspends once again. First polar body is extruded in perivitelline space during this process. This preovulatory oocyte nuclear maturation is accompanied by cytoplasmic maturation, which enables oocyte to be capable of fertilization. The second meiotic division is completed after sperm penetration during fertilization with extrusion of second polar body.

As mentioned earlier, the fate of a follicle is either way: it can develop to become a mature follicle which subsequently ovulates to release oocyte or as in most cases, it undergoes atresia. Atresia involves several stages of degenerative changes within follicle that greatly vary with the growth stage of follicle. Different stages of atresia are sometimes indistinguishable in primordial and growing follicles, although rate of atresia is much higher in these types of follicles. It has been observed that atresia of primordial follicles in yak is very fast and only a shrink oocyte characterized by chromosomal agglomeration and cellular pyknosis are the indicators of follicle atresia. Two stages, early and late phases are apparent in atresia of growing follicles of yak. Early phase involve shrinking of oocyte and condensation of nuclei, but without any noticeable changes in granulosa cells and basement membrane. Late phase of atresia is characterized by plasmorhexis of oocyte, with epithelial cells separated from the wall and coming into antrum to form a group of cells (Cui and Yu, 1999). The different stages of atresia of a Graafian follicle are well discernable and involve early, definite and late stages. Studies in yak showed that early stage of atresia involves three important changes within the follicle. First, loosening and sloughing of granulosa cells lining the antrum. Second, disappearance of membrana propria and loss of orientation of basal layer of granulosum and third, shortening and rounding of theca interna cells. Definite stage of atresia can be evident from collapsing, contracting or cystic signs within the follicle. Collapsing signs involves penetration of fibrocytes from theca interna into the granulosa layer. The membrana propria disintegrates invariably. This type of atresia is more common in cow and is rare in new born calves. In contracting atresia, the granulosa layers completely disintegrates and hyalinization of theca layers occurs. This is the predominant mode of follicular regression that comprises nearly 80 percent of all the definite atresia. Cystic follicular atresia occurs late frequently and is rare in newborn calves. Late atresia is the final stage of follicular regression. In this stage, the size of granulosa cells is reduced and the cell layers are completely disorganized. The theca layers are hyalinized. The antrum becomes gradually filled in with fibrous remnants of granulosa cells. Several factors, viz. age and stage of reproductive cycle, balance of steroid hormones, nutritional state of animal etc. are involved in determining the rate and stage at which a follicle becomes atretic.

A number of intra and extra ovarian factors, including steroid hormones are involved in regulation of follicular growth, maturation, ovulation and atresia. All cell types of ovary, especially granulosa cells and theca cells are capable of producing steroids. Appropriate concentration and an optimum ratio of steroids direct the fate of a follicle to become mature or atretic. FSH plays a major role in initiation of antrum formation in a growing follicle. FSH also stimulates proliferation of granulosa cells and follicular fluid formation. It increases the sensitivity of granulosa cell towards LH by increasing the number of LH receptor. The ratio of FSH: LH is also an important parameter for integrity and viability of the follicle. The current evidence suggests that the preantral stages of committed follicles are dependent on local regulators, with gonadotropins having a facilitatory role. The reverse is true for the antral follicles, where gonadotropins are essential for development, and locally produced hormones and growth factors play a facilitatory role.

4.3.4. Female Reproductive Cycle

Seasonal Breeding

Yaks are considered to be seasonal breeder and show estrous cycles only during warmer parts of the year. The onset and end of the period in the year when female yak come into oestrous is affected by climatic factors, grass growth and both latitude and altitude. At lower elevations (2400-2500 m) mating starts in early June and continues till late October (but occasionally into January). At higher altitudes (3000-4000 m), mating does not begin until mid-July and ends in mid-October (Sarbagishev *et al.,* 1989). Under Indian condition (2750 m), reproductive activity is at peak at July -August and lasts up to November (Prakash *et al.,* 2008). Variation in onset of first seasonal estrous has been observed at similar altitude, but with differences in air temperature and humidity. After August, as air temperature falls, the nutritive value declines as the grass goes to seed and then wilts. Thereafter, yak estrus decreases in frequency and stops around November. Recent studies on progesterone profile of yak, however, suggest that cyclicity could continue during non-breeding seasons also although animals may not show any behavioural symptoms of estrus (Sarkar *et al.,* 2006). Yaks kept in some zoological parks do not show obvious seasonality, possibly due to lack of seasonal variation in food supply. There could be a nutrition-reproduction interaction and seasonal pattern of cyclicity, as commonly observed in yak, may be due to an elevated state of nutrition during warmer months. During winter, environmental and nutritional stresses cause a severe deterioration of body condition of yak, which is reflected in poor or no cyclicity during this period. It is apparent, although not conclusive that seasonal breeding in the yak is determined more by nutritional status and dietary nutrition level than by photoperiodic sensitivity of the hypothalamic-pituitary axis. In general, cyclicity with behavioural estrus is seen in yak during July to November.

Estrous cycle

Estrous is defined as the time between periods of estrus. The events associated with estrous occurs in an organized and sequential way, except for periods of anestrus (absence of cycling) in seasonal breeders, as well as anestrus during pregnancy and the early postpartum period for all species. Yak females are seasonally polyestrous, although some cows show only a single estrous during breeding season and show estrous only in next year, irrespective of the fact whether she has calved or not. The average length of estrous cycle in yak is 20 days, although deviations have been noted in different conditions (Table 4.2). The detail of follicular, hormonal and behavioural changes associated with estrous cycle is discussed in the following sections.

Stages of estrous cycle

The events associated with estrous cycle can be divided into four stages viz. estrus, metestrus, diestrus and proestrus.

The estrus phase is characterized by high sexual activity, also called "heat", because it describes the degree of activity and excitement associated with this phase. This is the period when a female is receptive and allows a bull to be mounted. The corpus luteum (CL) undergoes full lysis and a new dominant follicle is ready to ovulate at this stage. During estrus, the vaginal and cervical mucus production is greatly increased and mucus may be visible hanging from the vulva or wrapped around the tail. Duration of estrus in yak female ranges from 9 - 72 h with average of 12-36 h (Table 4.2). It has been found that most yak start their oestrous in the early morning or in the evening and only rarely at other times of day (Lei Huanzhang 1964; Cai Li, 1989), although no definite trend has been observed with timing of estrus with other studies (Magash, 1991).

The period of metestrus begins with the cessation of estrus and lasts for about 3 - 5 days. Ovulation occurs during metestrus, about 28-36 hours after the onset of estrus. Time of ovulation in female yak vary greatly, as evidenced through different studies. This has been summarized in table 4.2. During metestrus period, the CL is undergoing early development. There may still be slight bloody vulvar discharge from some females due to the rupture of small vessels in the endometrium. Metestrus is period of formation of the corpus luteum. Progesterone levels are still low, but increasing slightly during metestrus. This is because the CL is small and does not have the capacity to produce large amounts of progesterone at this stage of development. During metestrus, prostaglandin F2α is not effective at lysing the immature, growing CL and causing a return to estrus.

Diestrus is characterized as the period in the cycle when the corpus luteum is fully functional. Diestrus, the period of the CL, starts about day 5 of the cycle and lasts about 12 days. The CL is producing increasing amounts of progesterone during the early days of diestrus, as the capacity for steroid production increases as the CL matures. During diestrus, external PGF2á can lyse the CL and initiate estrus.

Proestrus lasts about 2 to 3 days and is characterized by regression of the CL and the final growth phase of the ovulatory follicle. During this stage, final wave of follicular growth take place from where a dominant follicle grows from a group of selected growing follicles. As progesterone levels in the blood decrease, LH and estrogen positively feed-back on one another so that a rapid increase in estrogen production by the ovulatory follicle occurs, increasing blood concentrations.

Follicular dynamics

The number of ovarian follicles is predetermined early in a female's life. Although in yak follicular dynamics during estrus cycle has not been studied in detail, as like much similarities with bovine estrous cycle, ovarian follicles of yak are also expected to undergo dramatic changes. The use of real-time ultrasonography has demonstrated that development of an ovulatory or dominant follicle from the small antral stage during the bovine estrous cycle is characterized by a wave-like pattern of follicular development, referred to as "follicular waves". Each wave occurs in several distinct phases: "recruitment," the entrance of a cohort of small antral follicles into the acutely gonadotropin-dependent stage; "selection," a reduction of the number of recruited excess follicles to one follicle (future dominant follicle); and "dominance," the inhibition of additional follicular recruitment and development by the selected follicle, which escapes initial atresia and continues to grow until ovulation or atresia.

Initial Recruitment of a Follicle

Mechanisms for controlling initial growth of follicles have been difficult to determine and not clearly understood. However, there is a definite role of FSH in early follicular growth. Under influence of FSH, a group of follicles, all of similar size, emerged as a cohort. This cohort continues to grow during metestrus and proestrus, i.e. at the earlier stage of the estrous cycle (days 0-3). Those that are not recruited to enter into the initial growing phases are thought to be under some type of inhibitory influence keeping these follicles from growing. From this cohort a single follicle will be selected to grow further in pursuit of ovulating while the others become atretic. For the rest of the follicular pool, growth will remain halted until selected for initial recruitment and potential ovulation. It has not been conclusive which factors determine this recruitment process of a particular cohort, preventing others, but the numbers of gonadotropin receptors within follicle, stage of meiosis of oocyte and structure of granulose cells have been implicated as possible factors.

Selection of Follicles

After recruitment of a cohort of follicles, the selection process is initiated, at the end of which a dominant follicle is selected to grow while other members undergo atresia. The ability of a preantral follicle to become a dominant follicle depends upon several factors including its responsiveness to gonadotropins, production of inhibin and estrogen from a follicle, and feedback between the follicles and the pituitary. Initially, growth of preantral follicles is dependent upon FSH, as preantral follicles have low amounts of gonadotropin receptors. As a result, any decrease in gonadotropin receptor concentrations decreases the ability of the preantral follicle to respond to FSH, thus making it less able to continue development. Suppression of FSH leads to a negative feedback loop where inhibin and estradiol from the follicle feedback to the hypothalamus, suppressing FSH secretion and causing other developing follicles to regress through lack of FSH binding to the granulosa cells. During further growing phase of follicular waves a follicle is selected from the growing cohort of follicles to continue growing and become future dominant follicle. The exact mechanism that is used to select the future dominant follicle for continued growth, even during periods of decreased concentrations of FSH is sill not clear. Various features of dominant follicle such as its ability to convert androgens to estradiol that then feeds back to the hypothalamus and pituitary and diminishes the circulating FSH, and number of gonadotropin receptors have been attributed for this.

Deviation of Dominant Follicle

Once selected, a dominant follicle grows under endocrine control of the gonadotropins that cause steriodogenic activity in the granulosa and theca cell layers of the follicle. Typically, a higher concentration of estradiol is observed in dominant follicles, which allows the follicle to trigger all the physiological events required for ovulation. The deviation of dominant follicle takes place after the follicle attains an optimum size. As a follicle reaches the desired size for deviation to begin, the other subordinate follicles found in the cohort stop growing and begin atresia. This may be caused by the negative feedback loop by dominant follicle with the pituitary, causing an increase in inhibin and estradiol production which leads to a reduction of FSH. Further growth of dominant follicle seems to be independent of FSH. As the FSH concentrations fall and subordinate follicles begin to regress, the future dominant follicle acquires the ability to produce receptor for LH. By expressing this receptor the follicle now can use the LH circulating in the follicular fluid as a means of sustaining its growth, separating it from the subordinates. The fate of a dominant follicle is dependent on whether it is exposed to endogenous or exogenous concentrations of LH sufficient to induce ovulation. The absence of a preovulatory surge of LH results in atresia of the dominant follicle and re-initiation of follicular recruitment. Follicular dynamics in cattle indicate that two to four follicular waves occur during each estrous cycle, but actual number of follicular waves has not been studied in yak.

Behavioural estrus

Signs of heat in yak are less obvious than in other cattle. At the onset of breeding season, young male sometime follow and try to mount female herdmates, although yak females are not generally followed by mature male until they are in heat. There may be marked individual variation in expressing the signs of estrus. Unlike cattle, bellowing is not a reliable indicator of estrus in yak and in some herds, it may totally be absent in estrus animals (Sarkar and Prakash, 2005a). The most reliable behavioural indicators of estrus are:

i. Following and mounting by male yaks
ii. Standing to be mounted by male yak
iii. Frequent urination
iv. Raising of tail
v. Congestion and swelling of vulva

Mucus is discharged from the vulva in a majority of females in estrus, but a substantial proportion of female show scanty or no such discharge (Sarkar *et al.*, 2006). Daily milk yield shows a dip during estrus although this could not, on its own, be used to accurately indicate the presence of estrus (Cai Li, 1989a). Loss of appetite, restlessness and alertness are other indicators expressed infrequently by yak females (Sarkar *et al.*, 2006). The genital organs show marked pronounced changes than behavioural signs with relaxed and open external os of cervix, turgid uterus and ovaries having palpable follicles.

Endocrine Changes Associated with Estrous Cycle

The estrous cycle in the adult female consists of all processes including gametogenesis, folliculogenesis, ovulation, corpus luteum function, and steroidogenesis in the ovary. The estrous cycle generally is divided into luteal and follicular phases. During these two phases of the estrous cycle, complex hormonal interactions in the hypothalamic-pituitary- gonadal axis, regulates development and regression of ovarian follicles and corpora lutea. Endocrine and neuroendocrine mechanisms through positive and negative feedback regulate secretion of the GnRH, gonadotropins, and ovarian steroids. Tonic release of FSH and LH from the anterior pituitary occurs in response to gonadotropin-releasing hormone (GnRH) secreted by the hypothalamus. Pulses of LH occur in synchrony with pulses of GnRH from the neurons of the hypothalamus. Primary factors modulating changes in the pulsatile secretion of LH are the steroid hormones from the ovary that function at the hypothalamic-pituitary axis during the estrous cycle. The extensive feedback mechanisms by ovarian steroids are, therefore, associated with the neuroendocrine function of the hypothalamus and endocrine function of the pituitary to regulate ovarian functions during the estrous cycle.

Concentration of LH, estradiol and progesterone.

In yak, there are two distinct modes of LH secretion. The pulsatile or tonic mode of LH release is generated in response to pulsatile GnRH release from the hypothalamus. This basal level (=0.31 ng/ml) of LH is reached after about 4 hr. of ovulation and show a slight increase (0.44±0.05 ng/ml) at the onset of estrus (Sarkar and Prakash, 2005a). An increase in tonic LH secretion during the pro-estrous period results from an increase in pulse frequency. Pulsatile LH release prevails at all reproductive states in yak, including the period before, during and after the preovulatory surge of gonadotropins. The preovulatory discharge of LH is referred to as the phasic mode of gonadotropin secretion. In yak, this surge initiates around 3 h after onset of estrus and higher level (5.47±0.61 ng/ml) is attained at about 8 h after onset of estrus (Sarkar and Prakash, 2005a). During preovulatory surge of LH, the mean peak concentration has been recorded as 10.11±0.35 ng/ml with LH concentration ranging from 8.75 - 11.51 ng/ml. This surge of LH in yak lasts 6-10 h (average 7.25±0.55 h) and is primarily evoked and sustained by decreased progesterone and increased estradiol secretion during the final stage of the estrous cycle.

The main source of estradiol is the largest non-atretic follicle that under influence of pulses gonadotropins secrets this hormone. The mean plasma estradiol concentrations during different phase of estrous cycle vary significantly. The peak concentration is reached on day of estrus which then sharply declines to basal level at day 2-3 of the cycle. The mean concentration thereafter, is at basal level except a small increase between day 6 to day 12 of the cycle. The plasma concentration of the hormone starts to increase during late luteal phase until it attains peak level during estrus. During early and mid and late luteal phases the mean plasma concentrations of estradiol have been recorded as 10.39±2.52, 8.26±1.2 and 6.7±1.69 pg/ml, respectively (Sarkar et *al.*, 2006).

Even though the progesterone concentration in the yak is high during the luteal phase, progesterone concentration is not temporally associated with LH pulses. During estrus, serum progesterone concentrations remain at a basal level (=2 ng/ml). After ovulation, during early luteal phase (0-6 day) the hormone concentration (0.84±0.32 ng/ml) is slightly above basal concentration and increased (1.63±0.07 ng/ml) during mid luteal phase (7-12 day). The hormone concentration then continues to increase and reach a peak (3.67±0.99 ng/ml) during late lutueal phase (13-19 days), thereafter declines sharply to basal levels at estrus (Sarkar et *al.*, 2006).

4.3.5 Gestation

The gestation is the period that extends from the time of fertilization until birth of the offspring. Fertilization, fusion of male sperm and the female egg, to form the zygote, takes place at the ampullaristhmic junction of the oviduct. The sperm must penetrate two membranes of egg, zona pellucida and vitelline membrane in order to complete fertilization. Zona reaction, penetration of the sperm into the zona pellucida, is facilitated by proteolytic enzymes released from acrosome. The last stage of sperm penetration into the egg involves the attachment of the sperm head to the surface of the vitelline membrane. This activates egg from its dormancy and development begins. Following penetration of sperm, zona membrane becomes impermeable to other sperms, a defence process to avoid polyspermy, called vitelline block. The newly formed zygote starts cleavage, simple mitotic divisions of one cell into two cells, two cells into four cells, four cells into eight cells, and so on. The embryo then moves from the oviduct into the uterus at about the 8-cell stage. At this point, the embryo is free-floating within the uterus, and depends upon uterine secretions for nourishment. By the 16- to 32-celled stage, the cells of the embryo are crowded together into a compact group still within the zona pellucida, known as a morulla. Fluid begins to collect between the cells, and an inner cavity or blastocyst appears. Once the cavity begins to expand, the embryo is known as a blastocyst. A single layer of large flattened cells, the trophoblast layer, surrounds a mass of smaller cells which lie to one side of the central cavity. The inner cell mass gives rise to the adult organism, while the cells of the trophoblast form the placenta embryonic membranes. While the embryo is undergoing cleavage and blastocyst formation, the uterus is also undergoing changes which prepare the way for implantation. The embryo is said to be implanted when it becomes fixed in position and physical contact with the mother is established. The embryo remains in the uterine cavity and whatever attachment it forms with the wall of the uterus before the formation of the placenta is of an extremely loose nature. Subsequently, the fetal chorionic membrane has formed a fragile attachment with two to four of the cotyledons surrounding the fetus. Within a few days maternal caruncles and fetal cotyledons have become so intimately interdigitated that the embryo is being completely nourished through the cotyledons. As the pregnancy progresses, gravid uterus undergo a phenomenal changes. The size of the ovary and the oviduct on the side of the gravid horn is substantially increased. After about one month after conception, the gravid uterus started to increase in diameter and distinction at this stage could be made between gravid and empty horns. However, the maternal caruncles and cotyledons were about equally developed in both uterine horns. Thereafter, the septum dividing the horns becomes indistinct and disappears as the foetus grows. This disappearance of septum has often been used as a tool for pregnancy diagnosis (Yu *et al.*, 1993a). The gravid horn sinks below the pelvic brim after two months of pregnancy. In yak, the placentation is of cotyledonary type, as in cow. The cotyledons are formed by the union of chorionic villi from the extraembryonic membranes that penetrate into caruncles, which are button-like projections on the endometrium. The placental attachment is classified as epitheliochorial. Mohanty *et al.* (2002) studied the placenta and cotyledonary attachment in yaks. The average placental weight was 1.6 ± 0.5 kg and the total numbers of cotyledons in pregnant and nonpregnant horns were 45.0 ± 7.1 kg and 27.3 ± 4.1 kg, receptively. Total cotyledon area was 1494 ± 327 sq cm. The total area of cotyledon had a positive correlation with the calf birth weight. There was also high positive correlation of average cotyledon area with after birth weight and calf birth weight.

The gestation length of female yak is shorter than that of Bos taurus cattle. Average gestation length in yak is 258 days, although wide range of gestation length has been reported by different workers (table 4.4). It appears that gestation length is short when a pure yak calf is carried than when female carries a hybrid calf (Cattle X Yak). The longer gestation lengths for the hybrid calves are associated with substantially higher birth weights relative to pure yak calves. The sex of calf is another factor and longer gestation periods have been noted with females carrying a male calf.

Parturition is relatively easy in yak when they carry pure yak calves. About 2 weeks before parturition the sacrosciatic ligaments begin to slacken and the vulva to swell. There may be thin mucous discharge from vulva week before parturition. Unlike cattle, the hypertrophy of mammary gland is seldom until the last month of pregnancy. Before 10 days of parturition, the glands, however, become markedly enlarged and oedematous and are firm to touch. The teats are closer to each other and lengthen 1-2 days before parturition (Yu et al., 1993a). When the time for parturition approaches, the female yak looks for a sheltered spot, such as a depression in the ground or a ditch, at a distance from the herd. Typical behaviour of the yak during labour includes lying on her side and standing up again for delivery when a pure yak calf is carried. Normally no assistance is required during delivery process and the umbilical chord is broken by the act of mechanical stretching as the cow gets up or the calf falls down after delivery. Afterbirth is expelled generally after 4-8 h of delivery. Dystocia is a rare occurrence in female yak with pure-bred calves, but is frequently encountered in females carrying hybrid calves. It appears that the relationship of calf size at birth to maternal size may be a critical factor in dystocia. Such cows should be observed carefully during per-partum period and assistance should be provided during delivery process. The dam generally licks the newborn calf for about ten minutes, after which the calf attempts to stand up and suckle.

The endocrine profile of different hormones during gestation and peri-partum periods of yak females has been studied by various workers. The progesterone profile showed marked similarity with that of a cow (Yu *et al.*, 1993a). It is seen that both serum and milk progesterone levels gradually increase till day 14 in both pregnant and non-pregnant animals. On day 15, progesterone level in pregnant animals show a transient drop and continue to rise again from day 16 to reach a higher level at around day 19. This transient drop of progesterone level is absent in non pregnant animals, where after a peak at day 15, progesterone level declines to reach a level significantly lower than that of pregnant cows at day 19. Progesterone level drops again around day 90 of gestation, probably due to decreased secretory function of corpus luteum. It again reaches higher level on day 150, although not confirmed but probably with contribution from placental progesterone. An abrupt decline, thereafter, was noticed on day 239, followed by a more gradual decline to basal level at parturition. This level is maintained for 20 days after parturition.

The mean plasma estradiol concentration maintains a steady level (20-22 pg/ml) from day of mating to day 30. It drops to a nadir at about day 60 and then rise gradually to a higher level (46.64±11.70 pg/ml) on day 210. The concentration increases progressively and reaches a peak (551.4±70.86 pg/ml) on day of parturition. This is followed by a steep decline to a low level (17.84±6.63 pg/ml), which is maintained for 20 days after parturition (Yu et al., 1993a).

Plasma PGF2α level, after a very low level throughout the pregnancy begins to increase (0.73±0.16 ng/ml) day 4 prior to parturition. A steep increase is thereafter followed, to reach a peak concentration (17.16±1.31 ng/ml) on the day of parturition. The level then declines sharply after the day of parturition and continue to decline to reach a lower level (0.28±0.09 ng/ml). This lower concentration is maintained for 20 days after parturition with narrow fluctuations (Prakash et al., 2008). Similar pattern, like PGF2á profile, is followed by cortisol. Plasma cortisol level show an increasing trend beginning day 2 prior to parturition (2.36±0.65 ng/ml). Concentration then sharply rises to a peak level (26.65±5.28 ng/ml) on the day of parturition. The level then declines gradually and a steady concentration (2.36±0.25 ng/ml) is reached on day 3 post-partum and maintained for 7 days after parturition (Prakash *et al.*, 2008).

Table 4.4 : Gestation length of yak as reported by different workers.

Calf type	Gestation length	Reference
Pure bred calves	258 days	Denisov (1938)
Pure Bred Male calf	260 days (253 - 278 days)	Lei Huanzhang (1964)
Pure Bred Female calves	250 days (226 - 283 days)	
Pure bred calves	258 days	Dubrovin (1992)
Pure bred calves	259 days (228 - 280 days)	Katzina and Maturova (1989)
Pure bred calves	254 days (248 - 258 days)	Yu *et al.* (1993)
Pure bred calves	258 days	Joshi *et al.* (1994)
Cattle X Yak hybrid calves	270 days	Cai Li (1989p)
Cattle X Yak hybrid calves	276 days	Denisov (1938)
Cattle X Yak hybrid male calves	277 ± 6.2 days	(Zhang Rongchang, 1989)
Cattle X Yak hybrid female calves	261 ± 7.6 days	

4.3.6 Assisted Reproductive Technologies (ART) in Yak

The yak, under current production systems is generally considered as subfertile. Reasons for the low fertility are multifactorial and not associated entirely with brief period of seasonality pattern of breeding. Yak heifers attain puberty much later than cattle and usual age of first conception extend to 3 to 4 years old. Expression of behavioural estrus in yaks is rather low, and often the females have long postpartum interval. Silent estrus constitutes the single largest factor responsible for poor reproductive efficiency in yaks. Besides, nutritional and seasonal factors affect various reproductive processes in yak and could be limiting factors for optimum reproductive efficiency. Problems associated with poor production potential due to high inbreeding depression also make yak husbandry less profitable and contribute to rapid decline of yak population.

Considering their importance in socio-economic life of high hill people, and a steep decline in their population, yaks need much serious attention for conservation. Augmenting reproduction through recent biotechnological intervention is therefore, a prerequisite for sustainable yak farming. Previously, many of the successful reproductive biotechniquesof cattle have been attempted in yak, but with limited success. Recently, expansion of commercial yak production has led much interest and refinement of these techniques, both for research and increased commercial production. Most of these techniques swivel around artificial control of estrous cycle and ovulation in females, but much has been done on embryo transfer and semen processing technologies also.

Artificial control of estrus and ovulation

A variety of hormones including estradiol, prostaglandin and progestins, when supplemented from outside, can mimic physiological events in the cycle and thus can shorten or lengthen the estrous cycle. Basically, there are two different principles of artificial regulation of estrous cycle. The first includes control of life span of corpus luteum without accurate knowledge of follicular dynamics. The second and more recent approach involves the manipulation of both luteal and follicular dynamics. First principle involves use of a luteolytic agent (e.g. $PGF_{2á}$) for regression of a responsive corpus luteum or controlled supplementation of progesterone that expands the normal life span of corpus luteum, so that when the supplementation is withdrawn, animal response with estrus. The second approach combines use of a luteolytic agent along with GnRH for controlling the follicular dynamics. New approaches to the manipulation of the estrous cycle have been applied without impairment of fertility.

Exogenous hormones in various treatment regimens have been used for estrus induction in the yak with considerable variation in results. Different treatment protocols and their effectiveness in controlling estrous cycle of yak have been summarized in table 4.5. While most of the earlier treatments involve use of a single hormone for extending or shortening life span of corpora lutea, recent protocols invariably incorporate GnRH or its analogue for controlling follicular growth and ovulation. The use of recent protocols like ovsynch (Pursley *et al.* 1995) and heatsynch (Lopes *et al.* 2000) has advantages that treatment can be started on any day of the cycle and there is no need to detect estrus. This has immense significance in yak as expression of behavioural estrus is generally poor in these animals. In most cases, effectiveness of these treatments is measured by expression of behavoiural estrus or conception rate, which are compound physiological phenomenon and are perhaps, insufficient for providing accurate result. The development of yak specific hormonal assay is quite recent and has potential for providing an accurate response to different treatment protocols. In general, the results of these studies seem encouraging, although extensive research is further required before large scale application of these techniques.

Superovulation and Embryo Transfer

A number of advantages including the potential for producing more embryos from animals of superior genetic merit have made superovulation and embryo transfer programs more attractive for commercial yak production. Satisfactory responses, however, have not been consistently achieved, thereby limiting the use of embryo transfer in this species. Use of a progesterone implant (CIDR containing 1.2 g progesterone) for 12 days, with Lutalyse (PGF2á) injected on the third day after the first injection of FSH has been reported to have a mediocre superovulatory response (average number of luteal glands and follicles were 5.0 + 0.6 and 1.3 + 0.9, respectively) but no embryo recovery was reported (Zagdsuren *et al.*, 1997). Use of FSH and PMSG has yielded satisfactory superovulation rate in yak cows. The average number of ovarian follicles was 5.4 + 0.65 and 4.5 + 0.43 of them were found to be ovulated (Davaa *et al.* 2000). In a trial, cyclic yaks were synchronized using Ovsynch protocol. On day 10 after expected oestrus, animals received a total of 200 mg Folltropin, twice daily over 4 days. From 9 yaks, 27 ovulations were detected and 16 embryos were recovered (Sarkar *et al.* 2007a). In another trial, Sarkar *et al.* (2006b) used following protocol for superovulation in yak female: ovsynch protocol followed by Folltropin injection on day 20 after first GnRH injection, twice daily, equal doses, over 4 days period in association with two injections of prostaglandin analogues on 48 and 60 h after initiation of superovulation. The females were mated and the number of corpus luteum was recorded on day 7 after the last injection of FSH. The average number of palpable corpus luteum was 2 ± 0.71. In the same experiment, the researchers were successful to produce first yak calf through embryo transfer technology. Excluding this report, other *in vitro* embryo production studies have been successful to produce embryos that are capable of developing up to the blastula phase only (Chen et al. 1997; Luo and Yang, 1994).

Table 4.5 : Different hormonal treatment protocols for synchronization of estrus and ovulation in yak

Treatment regime	Estrus shown after	Synchronization rate (%)	Conception rate (%)	Reference
Two injections of $PGF_{2\alpha}$ at 10 days interval	3 days	82.6-90	77.9-78.9	Magash (1997)
"Three in One" Injection of testosterone propionate, progesterone, and estradiol benzoate	5 days	64-71	31	Liu and Shuai (1985) Shao (1986)
Single injection of luteinizing hormone releasing hormone-A2 (LRH-A2)	7 days	80	73.64	Wang and Zhang (1998)
Single injection of a combination of $PGF_{2\alpha}$ and GnRH	7 days	78.9	47.6	Wang and Zhang (1998)
Single injection of luteinizing hormone releasing hormone-A2 (LRH-A2)	1-10 days	80-95	86	Yu and Liu (1996)
FSH on day 0 and LRH-A_2 on day 2 (lactating animals)	1-10 days	70	73	Yu and Liu (1996)
Ovsynch protocol GnRH (0 day) + $PGF_{2\alpha}$ (day 7) + GnRH (day 9)	10 days	87.5-100	55-60 (Timed AI)	Sarkar and Prakash (2005w) Sarkar et al. (2009)
Heatsynch GnRH (0 day) + $PGF_{2\alpha}$ (day 7) + estradiol cypionate (day 9)	10 days	100	40 (Timed AI)	Sarkar et al. (2007)

The studies carried out on reproductive biotechniques in augmentation of yak reproduction have shown promising result. There are however, a huge scope of refinement and improvements. The current knowledge of basic patterns of follicle development in yaks is insufficient to develop and apply protocols for induction of estrus. The induction of estrus would be a useful tool to study the process and patterns of follicular dynamics in yaks.

References

Cai Bolin (1981). Introduction to the Maiwa yak. *Journal of China Yak*, 1: 33-36.

Cai Li (1980). Study on the reproductive organs in female yak. *Journal of China Yak*, 3: 10-16.

Cai Li (1989). Reproductive performance of yak. *Journal of Southwest Nationalities College* (Animal Husbandry and Veterinary Sciences Edition), 15 (2): 52-65.

Cai Li (1989a). Sichuan yak. Chengdu, China, Sichuan Nationality Press. 223 pp. In: The Yak, Second ed. 2003. RAP publication

Cai, B. L. (1981). The yak in Xiawa. *Chinese Yak* 1, 33-4. (In Chinese): In : Reproductive Patterns of the Yak. I. Reproductive Phenomena of the Female Yak. *Br. vet.J.* (1993). 149, 579-583

Chen JB, Hai LQ, Yi H et al. Comparison on effect on in vitro fertilization between the yak and ordinary cattle. In: Proceedings of the 2nd Int Cong Yak, China, 1997; 195-197.

Cheng WD, Liu Q. Studies on increasing the production of female yaks. In: Proceedings of the First International Congress on Yak. Lanzhou, China;1994, p. 309-11

Cui Y and Yu SJ. An anatomical study of the internal genital organs of the yaks at different ages. Vet J 1999; 157:192-196.

Cui, Y. and Yu, S.J. 1999. Ovarian morphology and follicular systems in yaks of different ages. *The Veterinary Journal* 1999, 157, 197–205

Das, B.C. and Sarkar, M. 2004. Training and collection of semen from yak bull (Poephagus grunniens L.). In: Proceedings of Fourth International Congress on Yak. September 20-25, 2004, Chengdu, Sichuan.

Denisov, V.F. (1938). Hybridization if the yak with Kirghiz cattle and the Schwyz. *Izv. Acad. Nauk. USSR (Otd. mat. est., Ser. boil)*, 863-878. (Cited from *CAB Animal Breeding Abstracts*, 7: 116-117.)

Du Fusheng (1987). Preparation of frozen semen of Jiulong yak. *Journal of China Yak*, 1: 15-18.

Dubrovin, A.T. (1992). Yak breeding in the northern Caucasus. Zootekhniya, No. 3-4: 18-20.

Hedges, S. (2003) IUCN Red list of Threatened Species. International Union for Conservation of Nature and Natural Resources.

Joshi, D.D., Lund, P.N., Miller, D.J. & Shrestha, S.K. (1994). Yak production in Nepal. Proceedings of the first international congress on yak. *Journal of Gansu Agricultural University* (Special issue, June 1994) pp. 132-136.

Katiyar RD, Sinha SB. Yak breeding and their health problems in Sikkim. Livest Adviser 1983;2:37-42

Katzina EV, Maturova ET. The reproductive function of yak cows. Doklady Vsesoyuznoi Ordena Lenina Akademii Sel'skokhozyaistvennykh Nauk im VI Lenina 1989;4:26-9 [in Russian] In: Reproduction in female yaks (Bos grunniens)and opportunities for improvement. Theriogenology (2003) 59 1303-1312.

Katzina, E.V. & Maturova, E.T. (1989). The reproductive function of yak cows. *Doklady vsesoyuznoi ordena lenina akademii sel'skokhozyaistvennykh naukim V.I. Lenina*, 4: 26-29. (Cited from *CAB Animal Breeding Abstracts*, 58: 352.)

Katzina, E.V. & Maturova, E.T. (1989). The reproductive function of yak cows. *Doklady vsesoyuznoi ordena lenina akademii sel'skokhozyaistvennykh naukim V.I. Lenina*, 4: 26-29. (Cited from *CAB Animal Breeding Abstracts*, 58: 352.)

Lei Huanzhang (1964). Observation on the reproductive physiology and features of yak. *Journal of Chinese Animal Sciences*, 7: 1-3.

Liu H. Quantitive determination of daily production of spermatozoa in yaks. J China Yak 1993; 1:34-35.

Liu ZY, Shuai WW. The study on yak's oestrus synchronization by using three-in-one-hormone. J China Yak 1985; 2:24-27.

Liu,, W. L. and Liu, S. Y. (1982). Some reproductive performance of female yak in our pastureland. *Chinese Yak* 3, 29-31. (In Chinese)): In : Reproductive Patterns of the Yak. I. Reproductive Phenomena of the Female Yak. *Br. vet.J.* (1993). 149, 579-583.

Lopes FL, Arnold DR, Williams J, Pancarci SM, Thatcher MJ, Drost M, Thatcher WW, 2000: Use of estradiol cypionate for timed insemination. J Dairy Sci 83, 216 (Abstr).

Luo XL, Yang YZ. Research on in vitro maturation and development of oocyte in slaughtered yak. In: Proceedings of the 1st Int Cong on Yak, China, 1994; 311-313.

Lu, Z. L. 2000.Reproduction and Conservation of Wild Yaks. In: Recent Advances in Yak Reproduction, X. X. Zhao and R. C. Zhang (Eds.) Publisher: International Veterinary Information Service, Ithaca, New York, USA.

Magash A. The Use of biotechniques in yak reproduction. In: Proceedings of the Second International Congress on Yak. 1997; P175- 178.

Magash, A. (1990). Statische Massmalen diagnostischer Zuchthygienemerkmale bei Yakkûhen in der Mongolei. *Wiss. Zeitschift der Humboldt-Universität zu Berlin R.. Agrarwiss*, 39: 359-366. In: The Yak. Second Ed. RAP publication 2003.

Magash, A. (1991). Ergebnisse von Untersuchungen über die Physiologie des Sexualzyklus beim weiblichen Yak. *Monatschefte für Veterinärmedicin*, 46: 520-522. In: The yak. Second Ed. 2003. RAP publication

Mohanty, T.K., Ansari, M.R. & Pal, R.N. (2002). Anatomical characteristic of placenta and its relationship with calf birth weight in yak. Proceedings of the third international congress on yak, in Lhasa, China, 4-9 September 2000. International Livestock Research Institute (ILRI), Nairobi. pp 404-407.

Prakash, B.S., Sarkar, M. and Mondal, M. 2008. An Update on Reproduction in Yak and Mithun. Reprod Dom Anim 43 (Suppl. 2), 1–7

Purevzav, Z. & Beshlebnov, A.V. (1967). Some data on the physiology of reproduction in the yak. *Zhivotnovodstvo Mask*, 29: 92-94. (Cited from *CAB Animal Breeding Abstracts*, 36: 302-303.)

Pursely, J.R., Mee, M.O., Wiltban, M.C., 1995. Synchronisation of ovulation in dairy cows using PGF2 and GnRH. Theriogenology 44, 915–923.

Qiu Zhongquan and Zhu Qimin (1981). Histological study on the genital organs of female yak. *Journal of China Yak*, 4: 25-28.

Robinson, G.W. and Hennighausen, L. (1997) Inhibins and activins regulate mammary epithelial cell differentiation through mesenchymal-epithelial interactions. Development. 124, 2701-2708.

Sarbagishev BS, Rabochev VK, Terebaev AI. Yaks. In: Animal genetic resources of the USSR, vol. 65.Rome: FAO Animal Production and Health Paper; 1989, p. 357-64.

Sarkar M, Borah S, Chakraborty P, Deka BC, Sharma BC, Duttaborah B, Borah S, Baruah K, Ramesha KP, Pouro chottamne R, Kataktakware M, Sarvanan BC, Sengupta DH, Das S, Prakash BS, Bhattacharya M, 2006q: Calves born from anestrus yak (*Poephagus grunniens* L.) using ovsynch and superovulation treatment. Zool Sci 23, 721- 725.

Sarkar M, Chakraborty P, Sharma BC, Deka BC, Duttaborah BK, Mohanty TK, Prakash BS, 2007a: Assessment of superovulatory responses in terms of palpable corpora lutea and embryo recovery using plasma progesterone in yaks (Poephagus grunniens L.). Res Vet Sci, in press.

Sarkar M, Meyer HHD, Prakash BS, 2006: Is the yak (Poephagus grunniens L.) really a seasonal breeder? Theriogenology 65, 721–730.

Sarkar M, Prakash BS, 2005: Circadian variations in plasma levels of melatonin and prolactin during breeding and non- breeding seasons in yak (Poephagus grunniens L.). Anim. Reprod Sci 90, 149–162.

Sarkar M, Prakash BS, 2005a: Timing of ovulation in relation to onset of estrus and LH peak in yak (*Poephagus grunniens* L.). Anim Reprod Sci 86, 353–362.

Sarkar, M. and Prakash, B. S. 2005b Synchronization of ovulation in yaks (*Poephagus grunniens* L.) using $PGF_{2á}$ and GnRH. Theriogenology 63: 2494-2503.

Sarkar, M., Dutta Borah, B. K. and Prakash, B. S. 2009. Strategies to optimize reproductive efficiency by regulation of ovarian function in yak (*Poephagus grunniens* L.) Animal Reproduction Science 2009. 113: 205-211.

Sarkar, M., Dutta Borah, B.K., Bandopadhayay, S., Meyer, H.H.D. and Prakash, B.S. 2008. Season of the year influences semen output and concentrations of testosterone in circulation of yaks (Poephagus grunniens L.) Anim. Reprod. Sci. 115: 300-305

Shao BQ. Experiment on the synchronization of estrus in yak. J China Yak 1986; 2:41-43.

Tian, Y. Q. and Zhao, X. X. 2000. Ovarian Follicle Activity in Yak versus Cattle and Buffalo. In: Recent Advances in Yak Reproduction, X. X. Zhao and R. C. Zhang (Eds.). International Veterinary Information Service, Ithaca, New York, USA.

Wang JC, Zhang XR. Reproduction Control in Animals. Anhui Science and Technology Press, 1998; 374-380.

Wolf, F. R., J. O. Almquist, and E. B. Hale. 1965. Prepuberal behavior and puberal characteristics of beef bulls on high nutrient allowance. J. Anim. Sci. 24: 761–765.

Xia LJ. Analysis on the spermatogenesis in yaks and comparison with common cattle. J China Yak 1990a; 3:12-17.

Xia LJ. Seminiferous cycles in yak bulls. J China Yak 1990b; 3:8-11.

Xia LJ. Ultrastructure of yak spermatozoa. J China Yak 1990; 3:4-7.

Xu Z (1991). Study on the histology, anatomy and reproductive function of genital organs in yak and their F1 hybrids. *Journal of China Yak*, 3: 18-21.

Yan, P. (2000) Male Reproductive Physiology. In: Recent Advances in Yak Reproduction, X. X. Zhao and R. C. Zhang (Eds.) International Veterinary Information Service Ithaca, New York, USA.

Yu SJ and Liu ZP. Use of exogenous hormones to induce estrus in yak. Int Yak Newsletter 1996; 2:31-34.

Yu, D. X. (1983). General condition of yak in Xingjiang. *Chinese Yak* 1, 60-1. (In Chinese)): In : Reproductive Patterns of the Yak. I. Reproductive Phenomena of the Female Yak. *Br. vet.J.* (1993). 149, 579-583.

Yu, S.J., Huang, Y. M. and Chen, B. X. (1993). Reproductive Patterns of the Yak. I. Reproductive Phenomena of the Female Yak. *Br. vet.J.* (1993). 149, 579-583.

Yu, S.J., Huang, Y. M. and Chen, B. X. (1993a) Reproductive patterns of the yak. III. levels of progesterone and oestradiol-17flduring pregnancy and the periparturient period. *Br. vet. J.* (1993). 149, 595-602

Yun, Z (1994). The relationship between season and age of stud yak bull in Damxung. Proceedings of the first international congress on yak. *Journal of Gansu Agricultural University* (Special issue June 1994) pp. 303-307.

Zagdsuren Y, Davaa M, Magash A et al. Superovulation in female yaks. In: Proceedings of the 2nd Int Cong Yak 1997; 193-194.

Zhang Rongchang (1989). *China: the yak*. Lanzhou, China, Gansu Scientific and Technology Press. 386 pp.

Zhang ZW, Han XM, Cui X, Zhang RC, Xu CL, Wang YC. Observation of estrus and parturition characteristics in Tianzhu white yak. In: Proceedings of the Second International Congress on Yak. Xining, China; 1997, p. 189-92.

Zhongxuan, D and Fenying, H (1982). Report of survey on the Zhongdian yak. *Journal of China Yak*, 1: 75-82.

Zhu XS, Li KL, Wang YY. Observation of superfine structure of wild yak, semi-wild yak and domestic yak using electronic microscope. J China Yak 1988; 1:11-16.

Zi XD, Zhong GH, Wen YL, Cai L. Growth pattern and meat performance of Jiulong yak. Forage Livest 1996;3:1-4 [in Chinese].

Zhang, Z. W. 2000 Semen characteristics and artificial insemination in yak. In: Recent Advances in Yak Reproduction, X. X. Zhao and R. C. Zhang (Eds.) Publisher: International Veterinary Information Service, Ithaca, New York, USA.

❑❑❑

Chapter 5

Nutrition

Introduction

It is a biological process of chemical and physiological reaction which transform feeds/ fodders into body tissues and activities as a whole. It involves the ingestion and digestion, absorption of various nutrients, their transport to all body tissues, metabolism and removal of indigestible materials from the body and assimilation of absorbed nutrients in the productive purposes. Feed comprising of water, organic constituents (carbohydrate, protein, fat and vitamins) and inorganic constituents (major and mocro minerals) in variable amounts which are called as nutrients. These nutrients are required for maintenance, growth and repair, production and reproduction and other body functions in adequate quantity. The objective of studying the subject is to provide all essential nutrients in adequate quantity and optimum proportions to all organisms.

To meet the growing demand of huge human population, it is necessary to produce more and more animal products viz., milk, meat and other animal products at a very rapid rate. In India, traditional management of yak has similarity to that of practiced in Bhutan, Nepal

China and Tibet. The traditional practice is based on exploitation of natural resources especially the grazing land in higher altitudes and community land in nearby villages. These are so many factors which can lead to increased animal production but one of the most important sector is nutrition. Animals contribute a lot to the increasing demand of human food by transforming the products that has little or no use in human diet and nutrition. They produce meat and milk which is neither cultivable nor suitable for growing in the field crops. Under Indian condition, the animals reared on agricultural by-products (straws and stovers), several unconventional feeds and tree leaves which are of low nutritive value. In this field of science, researchers have engaged in utilizing the crop residues and feeds of low nutritive value for managing the growth and production for better economic growth. For better understanding the yak nutrition, basic animal nutrition and metabolism of nutrients have been discussed with special reference to yak.

5.1 Classification of feeds

Feeds for livestock are broadly classified according to amount of specific nutrient they furnish into the ration viz., roughage and concentrate. Roughages are bulky in nature, containing more than 18 percent crude fibre (CF) and low in total digestible nutrients or TDN (<60 percent) on air dry basis, whereas concentrate contains less CF (<18 percent) and high TDN (> 60 percent).

5.1.1 Roughage

As earlier discussed, these are rich in fibre (form the bulk of ration) and broadly classified in to dry and succulent roughage. Dry roughages are comprises hay and straws. Hay is the green crop preserved green to reduce the moisture content upto 15-20 percent which inhibits action of plant and microbial enzymes. Legumes are most suitable hay making as these are rich in protein and poor in soluble carbohydrate, though cowpea and berseem are not suitable as these got hollow stem which prevents drying process. Non legume grasses are not good for hay making as these are not palatable, poor in protein, mineral and vitamins.

Succulent roughages contains higher moisture and further sub divided in to roughage of pasture origin, tree leaves, cultivated fodder, silage, root crops and tubers. Around 8.6 million hectares of permanent pasture and grazing land, out of total geographical area 328.8 hectare,

are mostly situated on undulating and hilly areas. This may be natural which includes grasses in the hilly region, continually grazed and is found mainly in drier tropics where rainfall is inadequate and soils are deficient in arable crops and cultivated pasture is mostly intensively and rotationally grazed or strip graze. In case of rotational grazing, the paddock generally subdivided in to 2 parts where the animals move in such a manner, one paddock is used for an interval of one week. The objective of this method is to maximize the availability of productive stage for livestock.

Nutrients varied in the pastoral grasses i.e., CP may range 3 percent in mature grasses to 25 percent in young and heavily fertilized grasses. CF may vary from 20-40 percent and moisture content may vary from 70-90 percent. In the hilly region where yak are reared mostly depends on pastoral grasses during summer months at higher altitudes.

Tree leaves : In most of the cases sheep and goats are fed with tree leaves, though cattle have also fed during lean period. In early stage of growth, tree leaves are rich in CP and low in fibre, in contrary, protein content decreases with maturity.

Cultivated fodder crop : Fodder crops, which are of good nutritive value and if sufficient space is there in addition to growing cereals food crops are cultivated for livestock. People reared sufficient number of animals for milk and meat are interested for growing fodder crops in some areas under Indian condition. Northern states grown legumes for livestock where possibility of livestock rearing is high and sufficient area is under fodder cultivation. Cultivated fodder may be classified in to leguminous and non leguminous fodder. Nonlegumes like maize, sorghum, sudan grass which are grown in kharif season whereas barley, oat, bajra, napier, hybrid napier, para grass and guinea grasss etc. are grown in rabi season. Nutritive values of these crops are not comparable to the leguminous fodder but higher than agricultural by products and crop residues. In the lower altitudes grasses like *Seteria* sp, *Panicum* sp *pennisetum* sp, bajra hybrids and legume like *Desmodium* sp in addition to the above grasses/ forages may be cultivated. In higher altitudes grasses like *Dactylus* sp, *Lolium* sp, *Festuca* sp and *Phalaris* sp etc. while legumes like Clovers and lucerne may be cultivated. There are a number of top feeds for yak in available in high altitude region which are *Artocapus* sp, *Ficus* sp, *Premna* sp, *Bohmeria* sp, *Reevesia* sp, *Castonopsis* sp, *Bridelia* sp, *Eurya* sp, *Ampora* sp, *Macranga* sp, *Aldizia* sp, *Bauhinia* sp, *Trema* sp, *Sauruia* sp, *Rhyngopticum*, *Osbekia* sp,

Thysoleuna sp, *Carex* sp, *Symplocus* sp etc are available which have been reported in National Research Centre on Yak, (ICAR), Dirang, West Kemang, Arunachal Pradesh.

Tubers and root crops : Under Indian conditions feeding of root crops and tubers to the livestock is not widely practiced among the farmers. Depending on availability of potato, turnip, sweet potato and cassava have been used by the farmers in various parts of our country. These crops are different from root crops nutritionally by having higher dry matter (DM), low CF and starch or fructan as the storage carbohydrate instead sucrose as the storage carbohydrate in case of root crops. The example of root crops are turnip, swead, beet fodder and carrot. Cassava is a perennial crop cultivated for its edible roots. This can be used upto 10 percent in the ration but due to presence of cyanogenic glycoside, it is not used in higher quantity and advisable to use after sun drying.

Silage : This is a fermented fodder resulting from the storage of high moisture green crops, under complete anaerobic conditions. The structure where it is preserved known as silo which may be of different type structure, depending on economy of the farmers and raw material available. Soluble carbohydrate and the moisture of the crops produce organic acid (primarily lactate, acetic and formic acid) which ferment the green crop preserved inside the silo. Graminaceous crops viz., maize, sorghum, sudan grass, bajra etc are more suitable for silage preparation than leguminous fodder as they contain higher soluble sugar than the later. However, legumes can be preserved as silage by sprinkling molasses solution on to it. Silage preparation is not very successful under yak rearing places in India due to its climatic harshness and suitable temperature for fermenting the material may not available, though not much exercise have been done in this aspect.

5.1.2 Concentrate

Concentrate may be defined as the ingredients that supplies primary nutrients i.e., carbohydrate, protein and fat at higher level, contain less than 18 percent CF and more than 60 percent TDN and nitrogen free extract (NFE). This may be classified as energy or carbohydrate rich which contains less than 18 percent CP and protein rich concentrates which contains more than 18 percent CP.

Energy rich concentrates : This is further classified as grains and seeds, mill by products, molasses and roots. Grains like maize, wheat, barley are major one and are used in feeding crossbreds of yak and cattle during advanced pregnancy and early lactation. Total digestible nutrients may vary from 72- 85 percent and CP may be around 8 percent.

Protein rich concentrate : Ingredients that contain more than 18 percent CP are classified as the protein rich concentrates. These are most expensive feed ingredients for livestock and incorporation in the feed must be economical from farmers point of view. It is established that in India, protein deficiency is more than 55 percent. These feeds supply essential amino acids and nitrogen (N) precursor to microbial protein in rumen. Protein rich concentrates again may be sub divided based on origin into plant protein, animal protein, non protein nitrogen (NPN) and single cell protein.

Plant proteins: Most important plant protein source for the animals are groundnut cake, mustard cake, linseed cake, sunflower cake but in Ladakh apricot cake is available in huge quantity and due to high level of cyanogenic glycosides, farmers are not using at field level as livestock feed. Mondal et al. (2011) and Mondal and Kakati (2008) evaluated this oilcake after detoxification by boiling in water for 1.5-2.0 h in broiler, Key Stone Golden birds, respectively without any adverse effect on growth, laying performance and slaughter traits. Similarly, the cake is being tried under field condition of Kargil for feeding to other livestock and till date no adverse effect reported by the farmers. In addition to these plant proteins are there for animal feeding but most of these are not being used in yak.

Animal Proteins: These are not used by the traditional farming community unless procured from adjoining states for poultry and other livestock. Most important is the fishmeal which contains around 50 percent CP with high digestibility value. Meat meal, bone meal, processed feather meal, blood meal may also be used in the feed but economy of the farmer must be looked into.

Non protein nitrogen (NPN): Ingredients that contain N in the form of amino acid, peptide, amines not the pure protein is called as NPN compound. This has got a special importance in ruminant nutrition as they can survive only on these compounds. These are successfully used under Indian condition with straws and other agricultural by-products, as crop residues are the main feed for livestock. Among the compounds like ammonium bicarbocarbonate, ammonium acetate and lactate, biuret and urea, last one is abundantly used by the farmers. Urea is cheap, easily available and contains 42-45 percent N, therefore the protein equivalent is around 250 percent. There are several methods by which urea can be fed to the ruminants, some of which are summarized below:

a. *Urea mixed with concentrate*: Urea can be mixed @ 3 percent maximum of concentrate or 1 percent of total DM in the ration. Urea must be mixed very well in the ration otherwise it will create toxicity which may even lead to death of the animals due to release of ammonia in higher quantities.

b. *Liquid supplements*: This is prepared by completely dissolving 2.5 parts of urea with 2.5 parts water, 1.0 part common salt, 2.0 parts mineral mixture and 92 parts molasses. The mixture should be uniformly mixed and the molasses is to supply readily available energy or more specifically the carbon skeleton for synthesis of amino acids.

c. *Urea mineral molasses block (UMMB):* In preparation of complete feed block for the animals, urea can be used with molasses and several minerals especially which are deficient for a particular area. Researchers are working in the field of mineral nutrition and to some extent they got some success to develop area specific mineral mixture. Research has to be conducted on area specific UMMB which will help farmers to nullify mineral as well as protein deficiency in livestock.

d. *Urea with crop residue*: In India, wheat and paddy straw production is more than 150 million tones per year. These are very poor in terms nutritive value i.e., it contains about 2-4 percent CP and 35-45 percent TDN. This is rich in anti- nutritional factors like silica (10-15 percent), oxalic acid (1.5 percent) and lignin which decreases its nutritive value. For feeding to the livestock under field condition, straws are extensively used. Urea treatment, one of the best method to overcome the situation have been adopted by the farmers. In this method, 4.0 kg urea in 50.0 lit of clean drinking water is mixed well and sprinkled on 100 kg of chopped straw. The treated straw is kept in a closed and anaerobic condition for a period of 7 to 30 days depending on environmental temperature. Within this reaction time, lingo-cellulosic bond loosen and hemicellulose available to the ruminants. Final product is air dried and fed to the ruminants.

e. *Urea mixed with silage*: Silage is the green fodder preserved anaerobically for lean period. Chopped maize fodder (30-40 percent DM) may be mixed well with urea @ 0.5 percent which will increase the protein value of maize silage. In some case, if it is added in a larger quantity, ammonia production will be high in rumen which after certain limit may produce toxicity and death. Chronic effect of higher urea feeding may be observed in milch animals as it may hamper energy metabolism, progesterone activity and embryo survival in cows.

Single cell protein: This is not used as protein under Indian situation for feeding to the livestock. Single cell organisms like yeast, bacteria, algae are cultivated in specilly designed ponds/ structures for multiplication of these organisms. Single cell organisms have special ability to grow very fast in a given period of time as compared to other organisms and researchers are exploiting these field for production of protein for animals.

5.2 Unconventional feedstuffs

India is facing heavy shortage of feeds and fodders for the livestock. According the researchers working in the field, more than 50 percent of protein and energy is deficit among the livestock. There is significant development of milling industry in terms of production of compound feed but not sufficient to fulfill the requirement. In most of the villages and hilly regions farmers using locally available feeds which are not available in other places or region are generally termed as unconventional feeds. These feeds are otherwise unutilized due to presence of one or more anti- nutritional/ toxic factors, though on processing of these feedstuffs can be utilized for feeding to the livestock. Unconventional feedstuffs may be classified as vegetable protein source, animal protein source, energy source and other unconventional feeds.

5.3 Functions of nutrients

Every nutrient has its specific functions to play in the body system. As we know there are six nutrients i.e., water, carbohydrate, protein, fat, minerals and vitamins and each of these have different functions, it will be discussed separately for each nutrients.

5.3.1 Water

Water is the ideal dispersing medium because of its solvent and ionizing powers which facilititates cell reaction and due to its high specific heat which helps to absorb the heat of these reactions with a minimum rise of temperature. Lean adult body contains about 70 percent of water, though the amount varies from embryo to mature animals. In case of animals, the water content is approximately 95 percent for of the embryo shortly after conception, 75-80 percent at birth, 65-72 percent at 5 months and 40-65 percent in mature animal which indicates the importance of water in animal body. Assuming 60 percent of body weight, intracellular fluid accounts for 50 percent of body weight, interstitial fluid about 15 percent and blood plasma 5 percent of body weight.

Sources of water: Water is available to the animals comes through various sources viz., drinking water, feeds and fodders, metabolic water, condensation process and preformed water. Metabolic water or oxidation water may be defined as the water produced inside the body by metabolic process which may be equivalent to 5-10 percent of total water and varies with metabolic rate. The following table shows the amount of water produced by different nutrients.

Bound water : It is combined with the constituent of protoplasm by either physical/ chemical means. It is very difficult separate from protoplasm by freezing at low temperature or by evaporation at high temperature under dry condition.

Water deprivation : When man is deprive of drinking water in a hot and dry environment, soon exhibits thirst. When deficiency comes to 4-5 percent of body weight there is discomfort, anorexia, when it comes to 6-10 percent, there is headache, lack in coordination, indistinct speeches, dyspnoea and cyanosis. At 12-14 percent level, eye sunken, skin becomes shriveled, there is inability to swallow and delirium occurs. Under hot environment, 12 percent deprivation is fatal to man. If water is lost from blood, its viscosity and the resistance to flow increases as result of which heart rate no longer be able to circulate blood fast enough to dissipate the heat from deeper parts and a fatal increase of body temperature occurs.

Functions of water

a. By solvent action, it serves as universal medium in which cellular reaction, ionic and other reaction takes place.

b. *Lubrication*: It act as lubricant to prevent friction and drying in joints, pleura, conjunctive etc.

c. *Hydrolytic action*: In this process H^+ and OH^- ions water introduced into bigger molecules to breakdown process.

d. *Cell rigidity and elasticity*: The body must have a definite form which it can be retain and yet within limits it must be able to change its shape by comprising to some extent to the force applied at any particular point. This is made possible by liquid content of the cell.

e. *Transport*: It acts as a vehicle for transporting absorbed and reabsorbed food materials and excretory products to the definite organ.

f. *Heat regulation*: As the specific heat of water is high, it is important in heat regulation of body by conduction and distribution, heat loss through urine, feces and respiration as well as sweating.

g. *Refractive medium*: The aquous humor helps to keep up the shape and tension of the eye ball and acts as the refractive medium of light.

It is therefore apparent that the animal should be given sufficient quantities of water. Deficiency of water if persists for long time, blood becomes thicker and body temperature rises.

5.3.2 Carbohydrate

Carbohydrate may be defined as the hydrates of carbon or polyhydroxy aldehyde or polyhydroxy ketone, their polymers and on hydrolysis produces monohydroxy alcohol or ketones i.e. simple sugars. Most plants comprise 60-90 percent carbohydrate and an adult human body comprises about 300-350 g of carbohydrate. Carbohydrates may be represented with a empirical formula $C_n(H_2O)_{n.}$

Classification : Carbohydrate may be classified into 3 major categories- monosaccharide, oligosaccharide and polysaccharides. Monosaccharides are simple sugars which can not be broken into smaller molecules upon hydrolysis. Disaccharides as the name implies yields 2 simple sugars upon hydrolysis whereas polysaccharides yields more than 2 simple sugars upon hydrolysis. Monosaccharides again, chemically sub classified into triose, tetrose, pentoses and hexoses. Important pentoses are arabinose (occur in gum, pectin etc.), xylose (derived from plum, cherries, grapes etc.) and important tetroses are ribose (found every living cell i.e. adenosine di phosphate or ADP, Adenosine tri phosphate ot ATP, riboflabin, nucleic acid of every living cell). Some important hexoses are listed below with their occurance.

Glucose : It is the major end product of digestion of carbohydrates by non ruminants and is the primary form to be utilized for energy in which these nutrients circulate in the blood of mammals. Glucose exists in the form of a pyranose ring and is more accurately depicted in the Haworth perspective (Figure 5.1). Depending on position of H and OH at C-1, this exists in two form i.e. α and β. α is the precursor of starch and glycogen while, β is the form for cellulose.

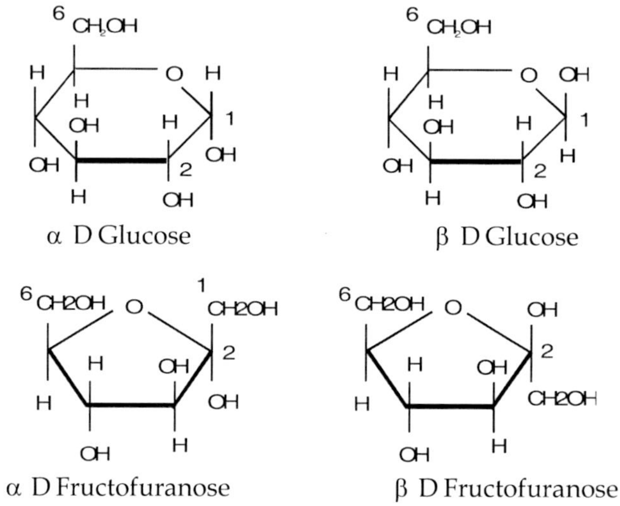

Figure 5.1 : Structure of glucose

Haworth perspective formulas of pyranose forms of D glucose and furanose forms of D fructose. The edges of the ring nearest the reader are presented by bold lines.

Galactose : It is an aldohexose which occurs in milk as a component an milk sugar- lactose. Certain compounds of galactose glycoside, occurs in brain and nervous tissue.

Fructose : It is the only keto hexose in nature and sweetest of the carbohydrate. It occurs free along with glucose and sucrose in honey, inulin is found in a number of plant where it serves an reserve polysaccharide .

Hexose compound : Glucose and numbers of other hexoses have the capacity to form amino sugars, several acids and alcohols. Glucosamine is an amino sugar in which one of the OH group is replaced by NH_2. It occurs in chitin, the shell covering of invertebrates, and is also present in saliva and gastric juices. Galactosamine occurs along with glucurnic acid in chondroitin sulphate a component the bile pigments which are important glucurmides.

Oligosaccharides : These compounds contain 2-6 glycose unit and accordingly classified as di, tri tetra and penta saccharides. Details have been discussed in tubular form (Table 5.1).

Table 5.1 : Various oligosaccharides and their occurrence in nature

Name	Particular	Occurrence
Disaccharide		
Sucrose	D glucose + D fructose	Sugar cane, sugar beet, ripe fruits, tree saps etc.
Maltose	α D glucose + α D glucose	Intermediate product of sugar digestion
Cellobiose	β -D glucose β + D glucose	Does not occur in free form, component of glucose polymer
Lactose	α D glucose + β -D galactose	Milk
Trisaccharide		
Raffinose	D glucose, D galactose and D fructose	
Tisaccharide		
Stachyose	Raffinose and D fructose	
Pentasaccharide		
Verbascose	Stachyose and D glucose	

Polysaccharide : Large number simple sugars are pohymerized to form polysaccharides which are of high in molecular weight and most of them are insoluble in water. There are classified as homoglycan those having only one glucose unit and hetero- glycan which contains 2-6 glucose unit, details have been shown in the following table 5.2.

Table 5.2 : Occurrence of various polysaccharides

Name	Particular	Occurrence
A. Starch	It exists in two forms amylose and anylopetin. Amylase is soluble in hot water, consists of straight chain of D glucose units in an α-1,4 linkages and the later is insoluble in water and is branched polymer of D glucose with chains of α 1,4 linked glucose connected by α -1, 6 cross linkage.	25-30 percent of most plant have amylose of total starch. Starch occurs in plants as small granules distinet in every plant and these granules are resistant to rupture. The granules on moist heating ruptures which is a irreversible change called as gelatinization.
B. Dextrins	Its defined group of intermediate of starch digestion and hydrolysis.	Dextrin favoured substrate for acidoplilic organisms in the digestive tract and when incorporated in the diet B vitamin synthesis in the gut is improved.
C. Glycogen	Its a polymer of glucose combined in an α- 1, 4 linkage and an α -1, 6 cross linkage. It has same molecular weight but side chain connsists of only 12 D glucose. Its water soluble gives red colour with iodine.	It is frequently called as animal starch and may make up 10 percent of wet weight of liver.
D. Cellulose	It is a polymer of ß-1,4 glucose. As such the 6th carbon atom are in *trans* position, which results in cellulose being flat band like microfibril. It is highly stable and fibrils held firmly by H bond and makes insoluble and resistant to microbial degradadation.	It is the most abundant substance in plant kingdom and major cell wall component and combined with lignin. Cotton is one of the purest form of cellulose.
E.Hemicellulose	It is not, as name implies, one half of cellulose rather a complex heterogenous mixture of mumber of different polymers of monosaccharide like glucose, xylose, mannose, arabinose and galactose. It is predominantly a xyloglucan. This is linked covalently to the pectic fraction of the cell wall and by H bonding to the cellulose microfibrils, thus adding to significant strength to cell wall.	It is also a principal component of cell wall and less resistant to chemical degradation.
F. Others Pectin, lignin chitin, plant gum etc.	These are polymers of vari ous monosacharides which are structural component of animal and plant cell and less important in nutrition.	

As far as nutrition is concerned, carbohydrate is classified into two major component-i.e., crude fibre (CF) and nitrogen tree extract (NFE). CF is determined by treating the feed sample with mild acid and alkali, whereas the later is estimated by difference –i.e., the equation after obtaining other fractions. NFE= 100 - (CP %+EE%+CF% + total moisture%). Due to some disadvantage to estimate by this method, Goering and Van Soest (1970) developed a method of fractionation of cell wall and correctly determine the fibre fractions and soluble carbohydrates in a given fed sample shown below.

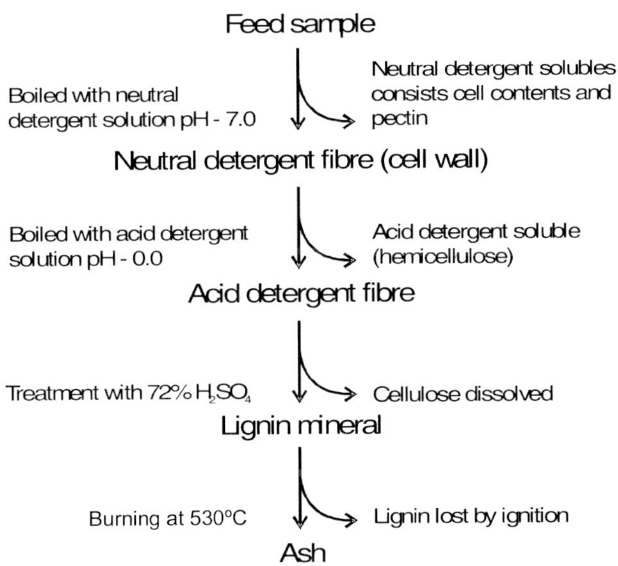

Figure 5.2 : Fractionation of cell wall components

A. Digestion, absorption and metabolism of carbohydrate in ruminants

As previously discussed that ruminant has stomach with multiple chambers and in the rumenoreticulum forages and other feeds are fermented by microbes.

Though bacteria, protozoa and fungi are in the ruminal content, the initial one plays the most vital role in carbohydrate digestion. The symbiotic relationship is developed to highest degree in ruminants as the rumen provides both the capacity and other factors which are most favourable to its activity. In addition to this effect, organisms synthesize essential amino acids and B vitamins. The volatile fatty acids are produced and various gasses are produced as the end product of different intermediately reactions. Carbohydrate of ruminant feeds like cellulose, starch, pentoses and hydrolyzed to monosaccharides by enzyme of bacterial origin and then fermented to volatile fatty acids. Volatile fatty acids mainly acetate, propionate and butyrate are produced in the ratio of 65: 25: 10 (though the ratio may vary depending on feeding practices of the animal), among which propionate is glucogenic and others are ketogenic. Depressed acetate production leads to milk with low fat content, commonly known as low fat syndrome found mostly in high producing cow and buffaloes. There is a change in production of these fatty acids that might be contributed by modifications/ alterations in feeding regimen. However, sudden change in roughage to concentrate ratio or shifting of feeding practices from dry fodder to green and concentrate to the animal has an impact on number and kind of microbes in rumen. There are several hypothesis/ evidence how carbohydrate is metabolized in the rumen but all agreed on the following simple reactions of carbohydrate metabolism in rumen (figure 5.3):

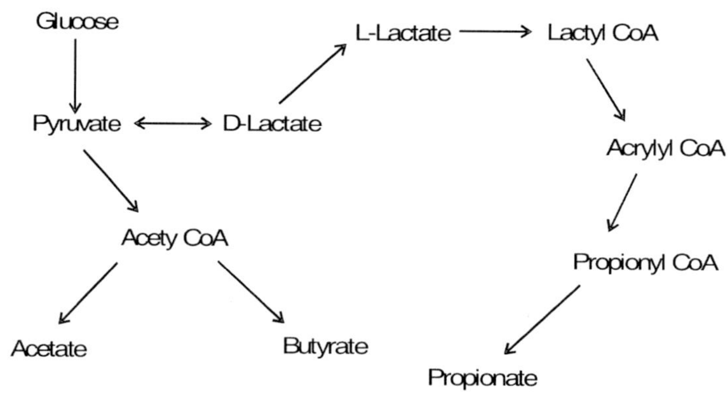

Figure 5.3 : Conversion of pyruvate to different volatile fatty acid (Hino and Kuroda, 1993)

It is important to indicate that if propionate produced from glucose via acrylate pathway, there will be less production of H_2, subsequently the CH_4. Fatty acids produced by microbial action are directly absorbed from rumen, reticulum, omasum and large intestine. The absorption from rumen is prompt and elevated levels of portal blood have been shown within 10 minutes after eating. The process appears to be by simple diffusion with the undissociated acid passing through at normal pH of 6.7. The rumen epithelium is not a simple sieve but has the capacity to metabolize VFAs as these are absorbed. Most of the butyrate is metabolized to ketone bodies thus portal and systemic blood almost devoid of butyrate. Around 50 percent of propionate may be metabolized to lactate and pyruvate during absorption.

Acetate largely passes through to enter blood stream and it is the only VFA found in peripheral circulation. It is phosphorylated to acetyl CoA and enters TCA cycle. It requires 2 high energy bonds to become activated and yields 12 moles of ATP upon oxidation. Thus net production is 10 moles of ATP. Propionate is largely removed from portal blood by liver where it is converted to glucose. It enters in the TCA cycle as succinyl CoA which requires biotin and cyanocobalamin. If propionate is converted to glucose and oxidized to CO_2 and water, net gain is 17 moles of ATP or 34 moles per glucose. Butyrate is absorbed as ketone bodies and eventually metabolized to acetyl CoA and net ATP production is 25 per mole. The glycolytic TCA cycle pathways are shown in the figure 5.4 and 5.5.

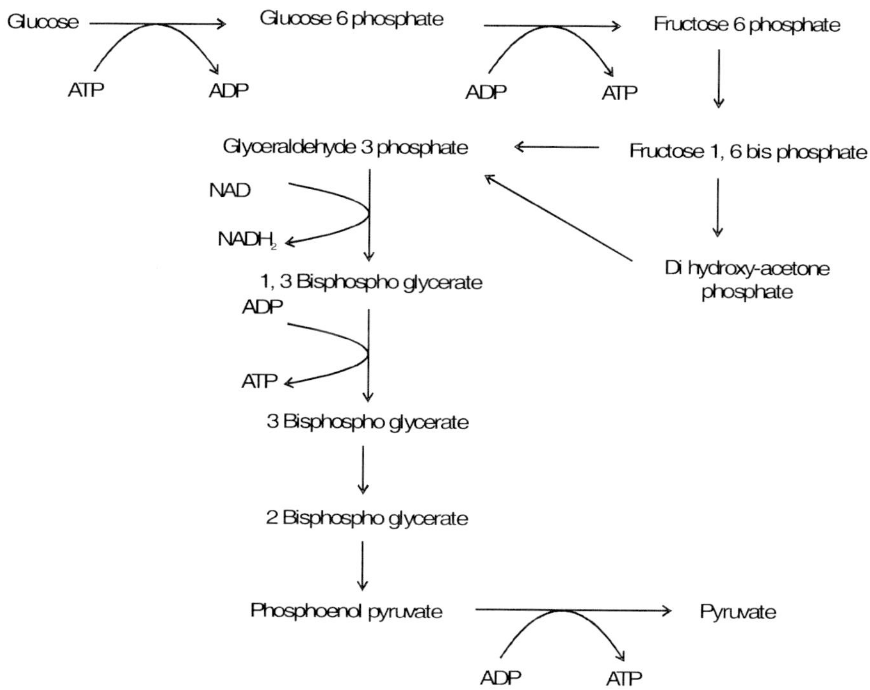

Figure 5.4 : Glycolytic pathway for pyruvate production

B. Supply of energy to the organism

The term energy originated from Greek words: 'en' meaning 'in' and ergon meaning 'work' and altogether 'energon' means active. Thus energy can be defined is as the force that enables body to carry out life sustaining activities. When nutrients oxidized inside the body, converted into mechanical or heat energy and chemical energy stored into feed/ food is converted from one to another. No function, not even body maintenance can be said to have absolute priority for food energy. A young animal receiving adequate protein but insufficient energy for maintenance may still store protein or wool growth continues while drawing on its reserve of fat.

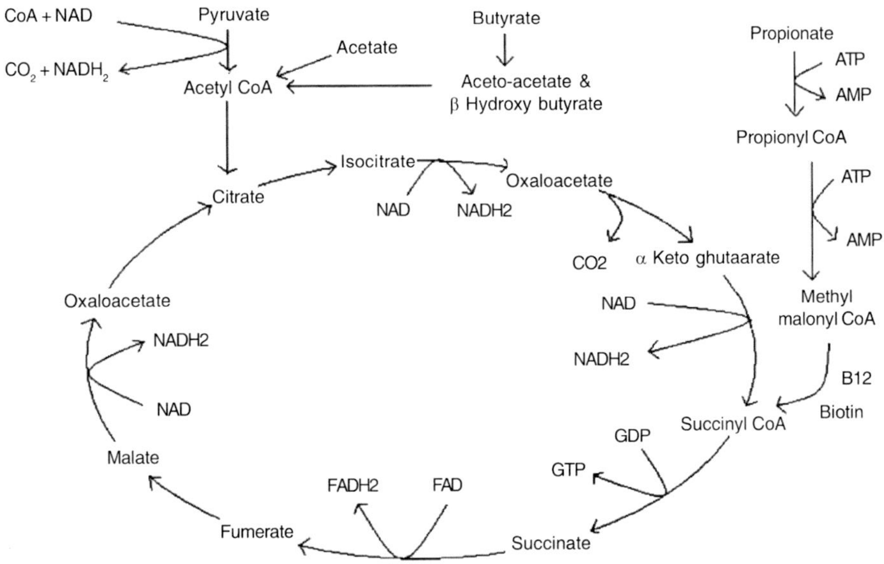

Figure 5.5 : TCA cycle/ Kreb's cycle and pathway of VFA metabolism ATP production.

The quantity of heat produced resulting from the complete oxidation of food is known as gross energy of that particular food or heat of combustion. This is measured in bomb calorimeter which consists of strong metal chamber (bomb) resting on an insulated tank of water. After placing the food material into the bomb, oxygen admitted under pressure and electrically ignited the food sample. Heat produced by the oxidation is absorbed by the bomb and the surrounding water. The quantity of heat produced is then calculated from the rise of temperature and the weights and specific heats of the water and the bomb. For carbohydrate, protein and fat the gross energy value is around 4.15, 5.65 and 9.40 kcal/ g, respectively. Of the gross energy of food, not all is available to the animal. Some of it is lost through feces, urine and gaseous excretion. Food energy that consumed less the fecal energy is called digestible energy. The sources of energy loss and utilization energy in the animal body is shown in the figure 5.6.

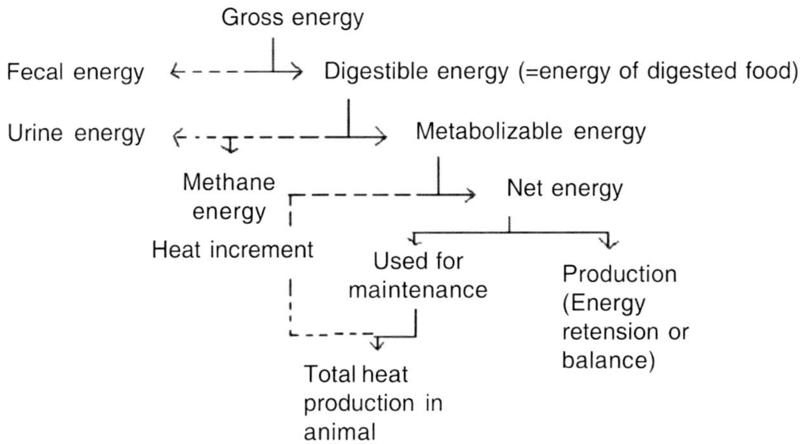

Figure 5.6 : The Partition of food energy in the animal (losses of energy are shown with dotted lines on the left side)

The animal suffers further losses of energy containing substances in its urine and particularly in ruminants, in its combustible gases (particularly methane) that leaving digestive tract. The metabolizable energy of a food is the digestible energy less the energy lost in urine and combustible gases. The energy of urine is present in N containing substances such as urea, hippuric acid, creatinine and allantoin and non nitrogenous compounds as glucouronates and citric acid. Methane production is closely related to food intake and at the maintenance level of nutrition about 7-9 percent of the gross energy of food. At higher level of intake it comes down to 6-7 percent of gross energy and it is possible to calculate the metabolizable energy of ruminant feeds from digestible energy value by multiplying 0.8. This implies that 20 percent of digestible energy is excreted through urine and methane. The ingestion of food by an animal is followed by losses of energy not only as chemical energy of its solid, liquid or gaseous but also heat. Animals are continuously producing heat and losing to it their surroundings, either directly by radiation, conduction and convection or indirectly by evaporation of water. If a fasting animal is given food, within few hours its heat production will increase above the level represented by basal metabolism. This increase is known as heat increment of food. In case of ruminants, heat increment has importance on utilization food energy on maintenance of body temperature. It is true that for maintenance, growth and milk production efficiency of metabolizable energy utilization varies from 40- 100 percent depending on type of diet and its digestibility. The deduction of heat increment of the food from its metabolizable value gives the net energy which actually used for production purposes in animal. Net energy used for maintenance is mainly used to perform work within body and will leave the animal as heat. That energy used for growth and fattening and for milk production, fibre production is either stored in the body or leaves it as chemical energy and the quantity so used is referred to as the animals energy retention.

5.3.3 Protein

As it is the principal constituent of the organs and soft structures of animal body, a liberal and continuous supply is needed in the blood throughout life for growth and repair, thus the transformation of food protein into body protein is very important part of nutrition. This is a collective one which embraces an enormous group of closely related but physiologically distinct numbers. Plant protein differ from each other and from animal protein. Each plant and animal species has its own specific protein, even in different organs it is specific one. The elementary composition of protein is carbon 51-55 percent, hydrogen 6-7 percent, nitrogen 15.5-18.0 percent, oxygen 21-24 percent, sulphur 0.5-2.0 percent and phosphorus 0-1.5 percent.

Proteins are the polymers of amino acid which vary in relative amounts and kind from protein to protein. These are the hydrolytic and enzymatic end product of protein. Amino acids are the derivatives of short chain fatty acids and contain a $-NH_2$ group and –COOH group. In acidic pH it acts as cation and in basic pH it acts as anion due to presence of NH_2 and COOH group. In the pH a particular amino acids act as electrically neutral and called as zwitterions and the pH is termed as isoelectric point for that amino acid.

Classification of Amino acids

A. Aliphatic amino acid

1. Mono amino-mono carboxylic acid (neutral)- glycine, alanine, serine, valine, leucine, isoleucine and threonine.
2. Mono amino-dicaboxylic (acidic) acid -aspertic acid and glutamic acid.
3. Diamino-monocarboxylic acid- lysine, arginine, citrulline.
4. Sulfur containing amino acid- Cysteine, cystine and methioine

B. Aromatic amino acid

Tyrosine, Phenyl almandine, Thyroxin

C. Heterocyclic amino acid

Histidine, Proline, Hydroxyproline, Tryphtophan

Classification of Protein

A. Proteins have been classified primarily on form, physical properties and chemical configuration.

1. *Simple protein*: Hydrolysis of simple protein yields amino acid or its derivatives.

2. *Conjugated protein*: When simple protein combined with a non- protein radical- called conjugated protein. Nucleoprotein, phosphoprotien, metalloprotien etc, are the examples of conjugated protein.

B. Structurally it can be fibrous protein which consists of a long chains of polypeptide and found in collagen and keratin. Collagen found as components of connective tissue and cornea. Its insoluble and indigestible but upon heating with acid, it becomes soluble, easily digested and the mixture of polypeptides called gelatin. It contains hydroxy- proline but devoid of cysteine or cystine. Elastin, part of tendons, arteries and other elastic tissues and found to contain cystine (22 percent).

Globular protein include enzymes, protein hormone and oxygen carrying proteins. These are soluble in water or aquous mixture of acids, bases or alcohol. Albumins are water soluble and are a significant part of serum protein and egg protein. Globulins are insoluble in water but solubility increases with changes in neutral fat concentration. Immuno-globulins and haemoglobulin in blood, lacto-globulins in milk, myoglobulins in muscles are some of the important examples.

Essentials and non- essential amino acid

Essential amino acids are those which cannot be synthesized in the body at a required rate by the body for normal functioning. Eight amino acid are dietary essential by all species and 10 are required by one or more species. These ten amino acids must be incorporated in the diet of most of the species and these are histaidine, isoleucine, lysine, leucine methionine, arginine, phenyl alanine, theronine, tryptophan and valine. Some of amino acids are synthesized inside the body, hence not required from the dietary source are called as non essential amino acid. Tyrosine, cystine, alanine, aspartic acid, glutamic acid, citrulline, hydroxy proline etc. are the example of dispensable or nonessential amino acid.

Digestion and absorption of protein

Yak is ruminant and inside rumen, bacteria protozoa and fungi play important role indigestion of food stuffs. The pathways how dietary nitrogen is fermented, digested, absorbed and metabolized ruminants including yak is shown in a diagramatic pathway (figure 5.7).

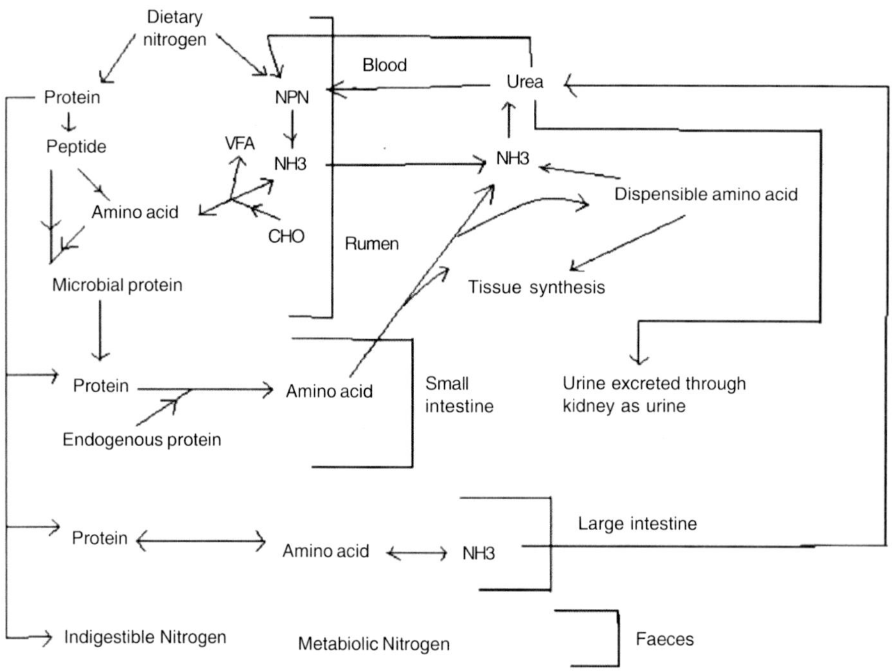

Figure 5.7 : Pathways of protein digestion and metabolism in ruminants

Some facts of protein digestion, absorption and metabolism in rumen.

1. Around 80 present of bacterial species comprising in rumen can utilize NH_3 as the sole source of N for growth while 26 present require it absolutely and 55 percent could use either NH_3 or amino acid.

2. As microbes multiply they synthesize protein to construct their own body mass obtaining the raw materials from ingested food. For the purpose microbes utilize amides, ammonium salt and other NPN compounds. Microbial protein synthesized in rumen, digested in abomasun and intestine, thus microbes play an important role in protein as well as carbohydrate digestion.
3. Amount of N recycled into rumen is around 12 percent of dietary N intake.
4. 40 percent of true dietary protein escapes rumen digestion and goes to the intestine while rest 60 percent true protein and all of dietary NPN along with recycled nitrogen contributes total ammonia pool.
5. 80-90 percent of all ruminal ammonia produced is incorporated into microbial nitrogen. When the ration fed does not exceed 13 percent dietary crude protein.
6. The rumen microbes synthesize all essential and non-essential amino acid for body building purposes. Hence the mixture of amino acids eventually enters the blood after the digestion of microbes and bears no relationship to the protein quality of original diet.
7. The digestibility of bacterial protein is lower (0.74) compared to protozoa protein (0.91) and thus, an net protein utilization is around 0.6. The biological value of the protein is 0.8, whether it is of bacterial or protozoa origin.
8. It has been established that for each kg organic matter digested in the rumen, 30 gm of microbial protein synthesized.
9. Sulphur, an essential mineral for microbial protein should be incorporated along with N in the diet with the ratio N:S is 10:1 (minimum).
10. Growth rate of microbes is greater than the flow rate of microbes from rumen to abomasums.
11. Rumen dilution rate may be defined as the proportion of total rumen volume leaving the rumen per hour and there is a positive co-relation between dilution rate and microbial growth.
12. Since the protein quality decreased in the rumen, in case of high quality protein feeds, bypass protein technology or bypass protein feeds can be incorporated in the high producing animals. These

feeds may be naturally occurring or heat, tannic acid, formaldehyde treated protein foods, using amino acid analogue or encapsulated amino acids.

13. With higher pH at rumen, NH_3 produced by protein fermentation absorbed at a higher rate and may cause NH_3 toxicity, in extreme condition animal may die, if corrective measures are not taken in time. Toxic level of NH_3 in rumen is 80 mg/100 ml rumen liquor.

14. For utilization of NH_3 by the microbes in rumen, molasses or other easily available carbohydrate is required as carbon skeleton for protein synthesis and energy supply.

15. For optimum growth, milk production and for higher growth and milk production in cow and buffalo, bypass protein feeds especially HCHO treated feeds are more beneficial than heat, tannic acid or lignosulphate treated feeds. Fibre of yak comprises of S containing amino acids and bypass protein feeds on fibre quality and production may be tried under cold arid condition.

Metabolism of protein

Liver is the key organ in metabolism of protein as it synthesizes protein, supplies amino acid to the circulation and processes nitrogen for excretion in excess. Its proper functioning depends not only its ability to absorb and retain amino acids but on its ability to provide judicious and carefully modulated release of them to the system.

Metabolism of protein involves few processes in the systems which are

1. Interconversion of NH_2 group (*trans* and *deamination*)
2. Synthesis of dispensable amino acid and other compounds
3. Amino acid for energy (gluconeogenesis).
4. Dispose of excess NH_3 or amino acid.
5. Catabolism of tissue protein and amino acid.

1. Interconversion of amino group

Transaminasion: This reaction occurs in mitochondria and cytoplasm of most cells in the body. It involves the exchange of NH_2 group from an amino acid to keto moiety of a keto acid.

Alamine + α ketoglutarate □ Glutamic acid + Pyruvate

Transaminase

Aspartate + α -ketoglutrate □ Glutamic acid + Oxaloacetate

The reactions are reversible and relieving NH_3 from amino acid to keto acid which enters into the TCA cycle for ATP production. Dispersible amino acids may be synthesized from glutamic acid and TCA cycle intermediates.

Deamination: There are two kinds of deamination- oxidative and non oxidative deamination in the system, of which oxidative is the important one. In this process glutamate oxidized to α-ketoglutarate leaving the NH_4^+ group and the principal enzyme involved is glutamate dehydrogenase.

L-Glutamate +NAD (NADP) +H_2O □ α -ketoglutarate + NH_4^+ + NADH (NADPH)

It is reversible, exergonic and dehydrogenation process. NH_4^+ released to enter urea cycle, whereas á -ketoglutarate can enter TCA cycle.

Non Oxidative deamination catabolised by amino acid dehydrogenase which requires vitamin B_6 as co-factor for completion of reaction.

Serine $\rightarrow$ Pyruvate + NH_4^+

Threonine $\rightarrow$ α –ketoglutarate + NH_4^+

2. Synthesis of dispensible or non essential amino acid and protein

There is almost 40 percent tissue protein comprises despensible amino acid. Not all amino acids are synthesized under normal condition as some of these are available from food in sufficient quantity. Glutamate, an effective source of non specific nitrogen synthesized from many amino acid reactions while, tyrosine and cystine are derived from the essential amino acids phenyl alanine and methionine, respectively.

Protein synthesis is one of the most important synthetic activities of the cell. It is said that in an adult human, over 300g of protein is synthesized a day. The high rate of synthesis give not only an indication of the degree of synthetic activity, but also point of fact that many amino acids are normally neutralized as a result of rapid turn over and recycling in the body. Protein synthesis not only literally mean deposition of new tissue but also the replacement of old one. This synthetic process require energy and it is estimated to be 8-10 high energy phosphate bonds per molecule of amino acid incorporated.

Mechanism of protein synthesis is very complicated and involving the role of de-oxyribonuclic acid (DNA) and ribonuclic acid (RNA) at cellular level. DNA serves as the template for synthesis of ribosomal RNA, messenger RNA and transfer RNA. These RNAs are all synthesized through a process called transcription by the action of an enzyme RNA polymerase in conjunction of with DNA. After transcription, mRNA moves to ribosome and paired with tRNA where sequence of amino acids to be placed in polypeptide chain and process is called translation. The tRNA released to be used once again and the ribosome moves along with mRNA molecule. Thus deficiency of just one amino acid would disrupt the process of protein synthesis and interfere with whole sequential process of biological activities of growth, production, reproduction and disease prevention.

Synthesis of special compounds

Absorbed nitrogen is used in the synthesis of number of special compounds required in the body process. Methionine, as it contains sulfur act as precursor of cysteine, hence cystine and taurine. Taurine is a component of bile acid as an excretory pathway of sulfur and the acid is essential for fat digestion. Methionine which has been activated to S- adenosylmethionine by ATP, serves as principal methyl group (CH_3) donor to as many as 40 different methyl group acceptors viz., creatine, adrenaline and choline. Tryptophan has a role to play in synthesis of special compounds like niacin. It along with vitamin B_6 acts as co-factor in many biochemical reactions.

3. Amino acid for energy

Unlike non ruminants, propionate acts as the main precursor of glucose and ATP in ruminants. As discussed earlier, any feed material in the rumen fermented by microbes and the fermentation product enters into abomasum and/or circulatory system for further metabolism. If there is deficiency of energy/ propionate in the circulation, fat and protein comes to play in production of ATP which is required for survivality of cell. Diagrammatic flow chart is shown below how amino acid enters in energy production in the system of both ruminant and non ruminants (figure 5.8).

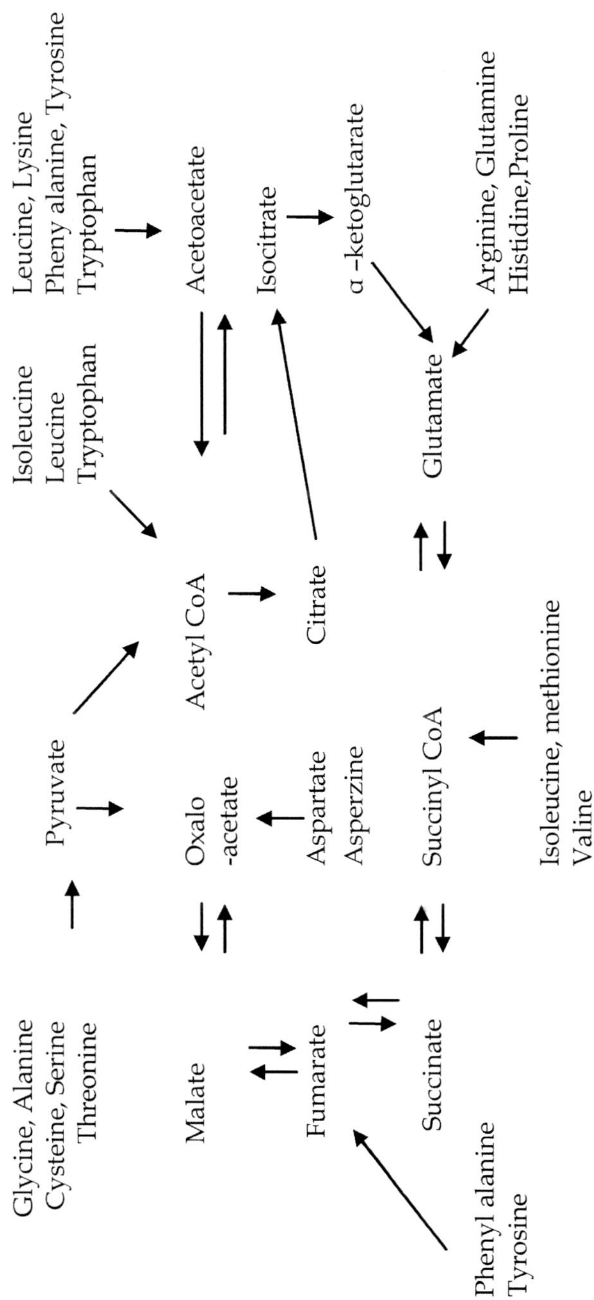

Figure 5.8 : Diagramatic presentation how the amino acids entering TCA cycle for production of ATP

Amino acids that do not enter at acetyl CoA in the process of gluconeogenesis and resulting in glucose production called as gluconeogenic amino acid. Those entering at acetyl CoA or acetoacetate can not result in net synthesis of glucose but could provide ketones and thus referred as ketogenic. Leucine and lysine are obligatory ketogenic amino acid.

4. Disposal of excess ammonia and amino acid

Most terrestrial vertebrates excrete ammonia in the urine as urea. Fowl and land based reptiles, because of limited water intake, excrete it as uric acid which is a solid. In fowls, uric acid is synthesized from glutamine, glycine and aspartic acid in a very complicated manner under the control of an enzyme xanthine oxidase. Most fishes excrete

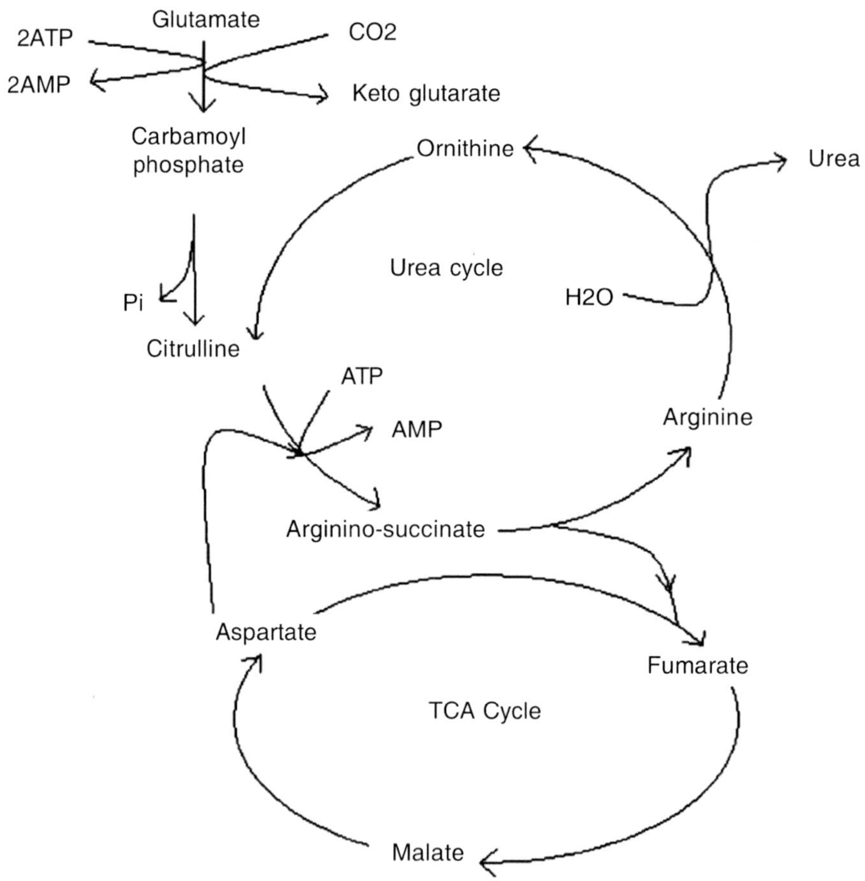

Figure 5.9 : Diagrammatic representation is shown below how urea is synthesized.

ammonia directly through the gill into their water environment. Ammonia, urea uric acid is the end product of protein metabolism and here we will discuss the process of urea synthesis as most mammals excrete it through urine. Urea is formed in liver in the urea cycle and excreted through kidney as urine (figure 5.9).

A total of three high energy bonds are generated and four are used up giving a net loss of one per mole of urea synthesized form glutamate. This has a special significance on post partum reproductive performance in animals. As animals are in negative energy balance following parturition and perhaps excess N in the food during the time, may aggravate the onset of estrous in the animal.

5. Catabolism of tissue protein and amino acid

The protein mass of the body, like adipose tissue, is in a continuous state of flux, with tissues constantly being catabolized and resynthesized. Rate of degradation and protein synthesis are regulated almost in the same manner and called as turn over. As amino acids released they become available to the general amino acid pool and can either be reused for protein synthesis or utilized as the source of energy. Two kinds of catabolism occur, that which is a normal function of tissue maintenance and renewal and that which follows periods of under nutrition. The amino acids have the same options for metabolism in either case but need of the animal dictate the route. Not all tissues have a similar rate of protein turn over. Renewal of intestinal mucosa is extremely rapid, 1-3 days in most species (Visek, 1972). The soluble protein of liver has a half life of 0.9 days while that in muscle is 10.7 days. Further the fibrous protein of muscle viz., myocin and actin have half life of 35 and 51 days, respectively (Maynard *et al.,* 1979). The shorter half life obviously reflects a more intense rate of degradation and synthesis. When a nutritional stress such as starvation strikes, tissue lost their protein and release amino acids at different rate as well. In general the integrity of those organs which are crucial for survival such as brain and kidney are maintained while liver rapidly losses tissue to support the organism. Muscle is somewhere in between. Thus on long stall feeding period or riding on high hills causes high degradation of tissue protein with lesser amount of synthesis, resulting in body weight loss in yak during winter months.

5.3.4 Lipids

It is defined as the substances that are insoluble in water but soluble in ether, chloroform, benzene and other organic solvents. This group includes the fat and a number of closely associated compounds. Fats or lipids play an important role in physiology and nutrition. One of the best example, we can say is cholesterol, which is the precursor of vitamin D and steroid in one hand and the infamous compound of atheromatous plaques of cardio-vascular disease on the other. It acts as the condensed reserve of the body, structural element of tissue and essentials of various reactions in intermediary metabolism.

A. Classification

It is classified as the saponifiable and non saponifiable fat. Saponifiable again classified as the simple fat and waxes whereas the compound fat as the glycolipids and phospholipids. Terpenes, steroids and prostaglandins are the example of nonsaponifianble lipids. Waxes are lipids resulting from combination of fatty acids and higher monohydroxy and di- hydroxy- alcohols. These have higher melting point and sufficiently difficult to saponify that these are not readily digested by animals. Common example is bee wax, a combination of palmitic acid and maricyl alcohol. Wax occurs as secretion and excretion in animals and insects and as protective coatings of plant. They are removed in the ether extract, thus, overestimates the nutritive significance of the assay.

Compound lipids : In biological system lipids contain a hydrophobic (non polar) end and a hydrophilic (polar) end which is essential for transportation. Examples of compound lipids are phospholipids, sphingolipids etc. Phospholipids consists of glycerol in which the 1 and 2 positions are esterified with long chain fatty acids. Saturated fatty acid in 1 and unsaturated fatty acid in position 2 , whereas, position 3 is esterified with phosphoric acid and turn to a nitrogen base. If the nitrogen base is choline, the phospholipids is lecithin, if it is ethnolamine, the phospholipids is cephalin. Both the lipids are component of cell membrane and involves in transport of lipid in plasma eg. chilomicrons and lipoproteins.

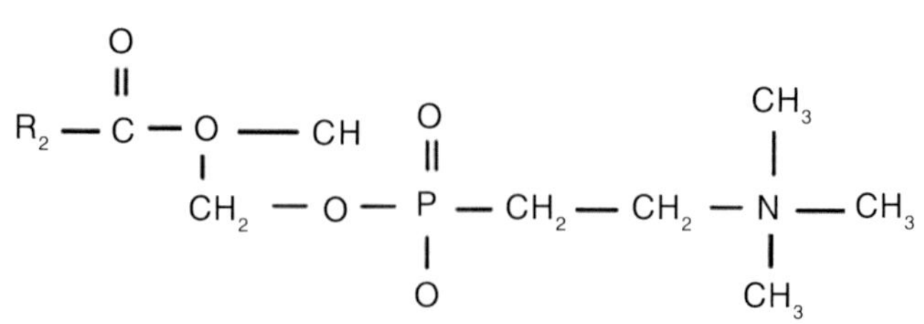

R2 - Fatty acid chain in the C3 position of glyceral dehydes

Shingolipids don't contain glycerol but consists of amino alcohol sphinosine to which is added a fatty acid phosphate and either choline or ethanolamine. In animals, these are found predominantly in brain and nerve tissues and called sphingomyelin. One special component of sphingolipid has the choline replaced with glucose and is called as the cerebroside, as shown below.

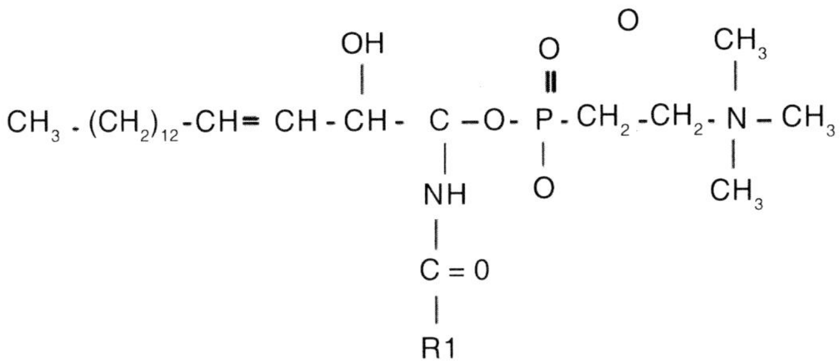

Glycolipids contain glycerol, with 2 poly unsaturated fatty acid joined to C2 and C3 position. In position C1, one or two moles of galactose is attached.

Prostaglandins : This group is non saponifiable and containing 20 carbon atom with cyclic structure between 8th and 12th carbon atom. These are found in almost all mammalian tissue and synthesized from linoleic acid. Their name comes from prostate gland, from where it was first identified. Though, recent advances of medical research shows that these are not confined to male genitalia but can be detected in several tissues of both sexes and are found to function as regulator of various tissue metabolism. These are often called as local hormone due to their activity within cells or nearby cells from where secreted. They work together with other established hormone to modify the chemical messages that other hormones brings to cell, though complete understanding requires research to conclude, even today.

From the standpoint of nutrition, it is the fact that main component of fat/ lipids are fatty acid. These are may be saturated and unsaturated fatty acid. Saturated fatty acids are those have no double or triple bond, on the contrary, the later have one or more double and/or triple bond. Polyunsaturated fatty acids have important role to play in various physiological functions.

Example of saturated fatty acids are butyrate (C4:0), caprioc (C6:0), caprylic (C8:0), capric (C10:0), lauric (C12:0), myristic (C14:0), palmitic (C16:0), stearate (C18:0), whereas the example of unsaturated fatty acid are palmitoleic acid (C16: $1\Delta^{9}$), oleic acid (C18: $1\Delta^{9}$), linoleic acid (C18: $2\Delta^{9:12}$), linolenic acid (C18: $3\Delta^{9:12:15}$) and arachidonic acid (C20: $4\Delta^{5:8:11:14}$).

B. Fat analysis and characterization

In routine feed analysis, lipids are determined as ether extract and it includes plant pigments, some essential oils thus ether extract in the feeds and fodder is not fully accurate which feed or fodder contains and available to the animal. There are some typical characteristics of food or feed fat required for routine analysis or identifying the origin of fat. Some of which are listed below.

a. *Melting point (or solidifying point):* Number of carbon atom when increased in saturated fatty acid, melting point increased, whereas, in unsaturated fatty acid melting point decreased with increasing carbon numbers of fatty acids.

b. *Iodine number*: It is defined as the number of grams of iodine absorbed by 100 g of vegetable or animal fat to be evaluated. It readily unites with the unsaturated fat at the double bond, two moles of iodine per double bond.

c. *Saponification number*: The number of milligrams of alkali (KOH) is required to saponify 1.0 g of fat is called the saponification number of that particular fat. As one mole of K^{+} reacts with each fatty acid, the larger the saponification number, the smaller the average chain length.

d. *Reichert- Meissl number*: The determination of the amount of water soluble, steam volatile fatty acid is a useful measure of the butter fat and is used for detecting its adulteration, since the high percentage of these acids in butterfat are its distinctive feature. This measure is called as Reichert Meissl number.

e. *Rancidity*: It may be of 2 type, viz., hydrolytic and oxidative depending on type of reaction with the fat. When unsaturated fat or butter are stored they become rancid due to hydrolytic activity of the microbes. These secrete lipase which splits triglyceride to mono and di- glyceride, glycerol and free fatty acid. Low molecular fatty acids give bad flavour and odour to the particular fat. This type of rancidity can be reduced by refrigeration, exclusion of water or by destroying hydrolytic microbes. In case of oxidative rancidity, hydrogen, oxygen and halogens are combined with unsaturated fatty acids. This reaction of hydrogen with fats and oils is used commercially to produce hydrogenated fats.

C. Digestion, absorption and metabolism of fat

Ruminants has the four compartment stomach viz., rumen, reticulum, omasum and abomasum. In the young suckling calves rumen not developed and digestion takes place like the non ruminants. Rumen develops between 8- 12 weeks of age and until then enzymatic digestion takes place. After the period, ruminal fermentation occurs in rumen and along with digesta and microbe flushed to true stomach or abomasum, which subsequently digested enzymatically like other non- ruminants. The factors which are responsible for the fermentation of food are slow passage of ingesta, buffering action saliva, continuous removal of soluble products etc which favoured by the unique activity of ruminal microbes.

Fats are hydrolyzed to fatty acid and glycerol by ruminal microbes. The mixed bacterial population is responsible for fat hydrolysis and hydrogenation. *Anaerovibrio lipolytica* are known to its activity in fat fermentation in rumen, though other bacteria, protozoa and fungi have some role in fat hydrolysis and hydrogenation in rumen. The end product of hydrolysis and hydrogenation are either taken up by microbes or flushed out to the lower gut where lipase acts on it for absorption. The possible pathway of fat digestion is shown in figure 5.10.

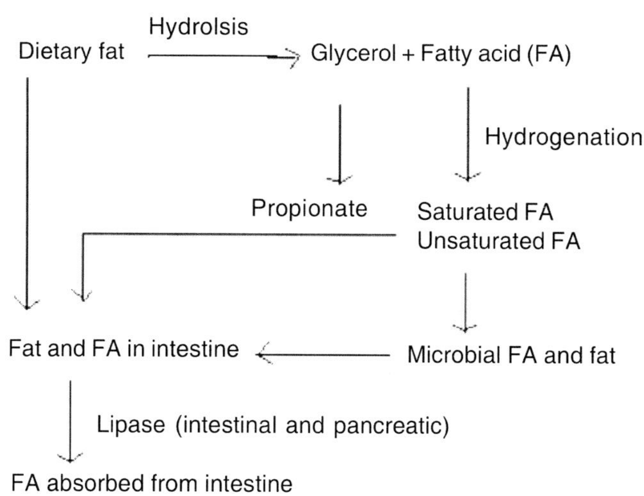

Figure 5.10 : Fat digestion in ruminants

Fat metabolism in ruminants: Most of the dietary lipids enter the lacteals as chylomicrons, free fatty acid and glycerol resulting from the complete hydrolysis of triglycerides. Liver is the key organ in both transport and utilization of triglycerides. The blood lipid rises due to intestinal absorption of dietary lipids, mobilization of stored fat or may come from synthetic processes in liver. The characteristics of blood lipid depends on so many factors like species, quality and quantity of dietary fat, age, hormonal balance and energy needs etc. In this regard it is to be noted that the triglyceride one of the most culprit in producing heart diseases in human beings, recently studied in detail and increased due to change in life style. However, glycerol and fatty acid metabolized in different way and again when required synthesized to fat or triglyceride. The oxidation of fatty acids is the step wise process involving cleavage of 2 carbon fragments starting from the carboxyl end of the chain. The process is called β oxidation. The intermediates in the fatty acid oxidation are all acyl (R-C-S-CoA) derivative of coenzyme. The net result of β oxidation is the production of acetyl CoA molecules. These molecule enter the Kreb cycle or TCA cycle and oxidized to CO_2 and water with the production of ATP. The glycerol is first converted to dihydroxy acetone phosphate which is then converted to acetyl CoA, then into Krebs cycle. The pathway of β oxidation is shown how in 4 step reaction 1 acetyl CoA released (figure 5.11).

D. Fat synthesis

When fatty acid oxidation was found to occur by oxidative removal of successive 2 carbon (acetyl CoA) units, biosynthesis of fatty acids catalyzed by different sets of enzyme and take place in various pars of cell. Moreover, a three carbon intermediate, malonyl CoA, participates in the synthetic pathway but not in their breakdown process.

The basic reaction sequence by which the long chains of carbon atom in fatty acid are assembled consists of 4 steps. The saturated acyl group produced during this set of reactions is recycled to become the substrate in another condensation process with an activated malonyl group. With each passage through the cycle, the fatty acyl chain is extended by two carbons. When the chain length reaches to 16 (palmitate) the product leaves the cycle. The methyl and carboxyl carbon atoms of the acetyl group become C16 and C15, respectively, of the end product i.e. palmitate. The rest of the carbon atoms are derived from malonyl CoA.

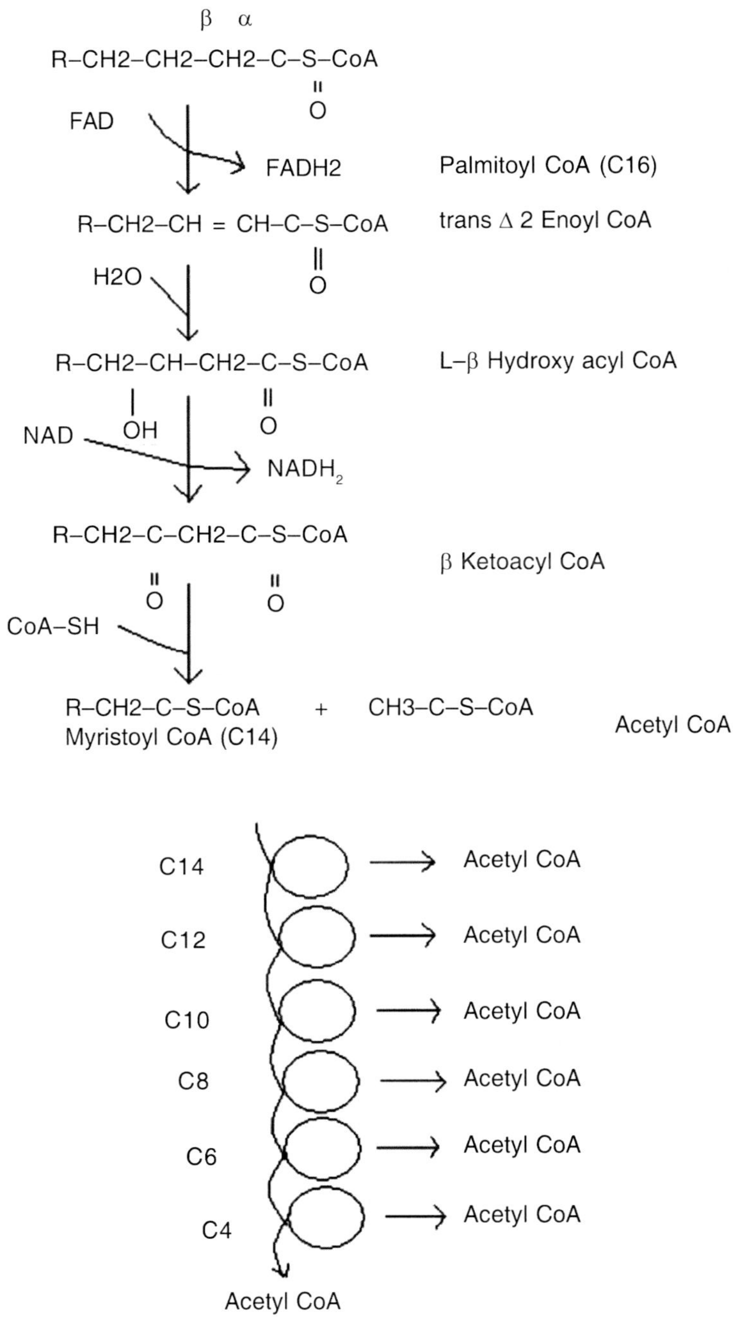

Figure 5.11 : The fatty acid oxidation pathway (basic 4 steps by which one acetyl CoA released initially and six more such passes through to yield seven more acetyl CoA. A total of 8 molecules of acetyl CoA are formed in all)

All the four steps reaction in the synthetic process are catalyzed by a multi-enzyme complex, fatty acid synthase, consists of 7 separate polypeptides and performs separate functions. Its location in the cell differ from one species to another but the reaction sequence is identical to all organisms. In addition to the enzyme complex, acyl carrier protein also plays an important role in fatty acid synthesis. Its a small protein containing prosthetic group 4/ phosphopentatheine and intermediate in the synthesis of CoA. The 4/ phosphopentatheine prosthetic group of acyl carrier protein (ACP) is believed to serve as a flexible arm, tethering the growing acyl chain to the surface of the fatty acid synthase complex and carrying the reaction intermediates from one enzyme active site to the next. Among the 4 step reaction, first (condensation) malonyl group and acetyl group condenses by removal of CO_2 from malonyl group and in the second step (reduction), C=O group reduced by accepting protons from NADPH + H^+. In the third step, H_2O is removed from (dehydration) acetyl group and in the last step acetyl group is again reduced (reduction) with the formation of saturated acyl group lengthened by 2 carbons. The same process is going on until the chain length reaches 16 and the enzyme system leaves the fatty acid. This is the precursor of other long chain fatty acid through the action of fatty acid elongation system which is present in smooth endoplasmic reticulum and mitochondria.

Synthesis of triglyceride : Most of the fatty acids are synthesized or ingested by an organism one of two fates: incorporation into triglycerides for storage of metabolic energy or incorporation in to the phospholipids of membrane. Partitioning between two alternatives depends on requirement of the organism. Animals can synthesize and store large quantity of triglyceride, to be used as fuel later. Whenever, carbohydrate is ingested in excess of the capacity to store glycogen, it is converted in to triglyceride as an energy rich fuel, stored in fruit, nuts and seeds. Triglycerols, and glycerophospholipids such as phosphatidylethanolamine share two precursors (fatty acyl CoA and glycerol 3 phosphate) and several enzymatic steps in their synthesis in the animal tussues. The steps are shown below how triglyceride is formed in animal body (figure 5.12).

The biosynthesis and degradation of triacylglycerols are regulated reciprocally with the favoured path depending on metabolic resource and need of that period/ moment. The rate of triglyceride biosynthesis is profoundly altered by the action of several hormones. Important one is insulin which converts carbohydrate in to triglycerides in two steps. In deficiency of or secretion failure of insulin, individual can not use glucose properly and fail to synthesize fatty acid from carbohydrate and amino acid. They increased rate of fat oxidation and ketone bodies with the consequence of loss of body weight. Triglyceride metabolism also influenced by glucagon, somatotropic hormone and adrenal cortical hormone etc.

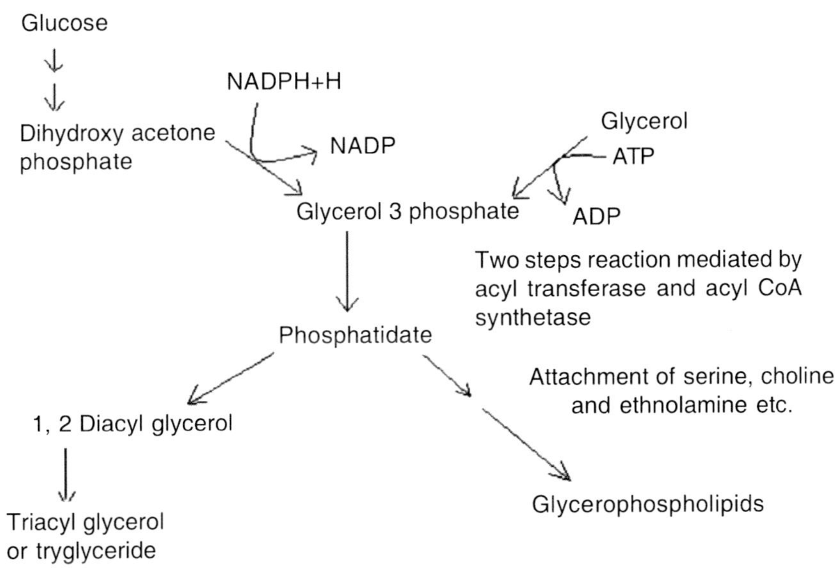

Figure 5.12 : Biosynthesis of triglycerides

5.3.5 Minerals

There are immensely important elements which require for various life processes as they are the basic component of all forms of life. Large number of elements of the periodic table has been found to be present in living cells but so far 25 minerals have been found to be dietary essential on the basis of there proven role in various metabolic role in the animal body. These are required in very small quantity as compared to carbohydrate, protein, fat, and water but deficiency may cause harmful effect in the body and some time may lead to death of the animals.

Classification

Depending on requirement of animal the minerals are classified in to two major classes viz., major or macro and micro or trace minerals. There are 7 minerals viz., Ca, P, Mg, S, Na, K and Cl are termed as major as these are needed in relatively higher quantity (i.e. in grams) and rests viz., Cu, Co, Zn, Fe, I, F, Mn, Ni, Si, Sn, V, Cd, Hg, Pb, Cr, As, Sc and Se are termed as trace mineral as these are needed relatively lower quantity (in microgram or even less) for large ruminants. In addition to these listed minerals there are 30 or so minerals that are needed for normal functioning of the animal body but exact role yet to be established.

Most of the minerals are distributed throughout the body where they exist in variety of functional combination and in characteristic concentrations which must be maintained within quite narrow limits if the functional and structural integrity of the tissue is to be safeguarded and the growth, health and productivity of the animal are to remain unimpaired. Continued ingestion of diets, that are deficient, imbalanced or excessively high in a particular element invariably induce changes in the functioning forms, activities or concentration of that element in the body tissues or fluids. Under these circumstances, biochemical defects develop, physiological functions are affected and structural disorders may arise in ways which vary with different elements, with the degree and duration of the dietary deficiency or toxicity and with age, sex and species of animal involved. However, there is generally a varying degree of gap between the essential and apparently toxic levels of intake.

Distribution

All the mineral elements have varying degree of distribution in plants and soil. Low or excess content of the element in plants and soil leads to the area problem of either deficiency or toxicity. Certain elements are antagonistic to each other while few plant species can accumulate high contents irrespective of their concentration in the soil and thus aggravate problems in the animals. Recent advances in agricultural practices viz., high yields of crop are likely to reduce the soil reserve of elements. In soils where total amount of available supplies is low, deficiencies will necessarily be greater. Changing crop pattern and fertilizers used have also been found to create imbalances of trace elements in soil, plants and animals. The leguminous fodder like berseem, alfalfa and cowpea contain adequate amounts of Cu, Fe, Mn and Zn. However, a wide variation in the content of these elements exists not only in from area to area but even in the fodders of the same area. There are several factors which affect the mineral distribution in plant. The major factors affecting the mineral content of crops and forage plants are those involving genetics of the plant, soil where the plants are grown, climate and weather, stage of maturity and the part of the plant. The above factors are interrelated in many ways. For example, often the climate has a major effect on the soil characteristics. In turn, the soil and climate often play important or decisive role in the type of plants grown.

Bioavailability of minerals

Bioavailability of any mineral relates to the degree to which an ingested mineral is absorbed and so is available to the body of the animal. While minerals are present in a feed, they are not available unless the body can absorb and utilize them. The ability to absorb minerals from a diet depends on many factors. A value listed in the feed composition table is just a starting point for estimating the true contribution a feed makes to the animals' mineral needs. Bioavailability in true sense, therefore, could be defined as the proportion of an ingested element i.e. absorbed, transported to the site of action and converted to the physiologically active species. There are several intrinsic and extrinsic factors which are affecting the bioavailability of minerals in the body.

The intrinsic factors are

a. Species and genotype
b. Age
c. Sex
d. Metabolic function i.e. maintenance, growth, reproduction/ lactation
e. Nutritional status including adaptation to dietary intake
f. Physiological stress
g. Intestinal microflora and infection

The extrinsic factors are

a. Solubility of the element species or form of mineral eg. CuS, $CuMnS_4$ and $Fe_4(P_2O_4)_3$
b. Adsorption of diet component on large surfaces eg. fibre, silica and $Ca_3(PO_4)_2$
c. State of oxidation of element; chemical form eg. Fe^{2+} vs. Fe^{3+}
d. Competitive antagonism between and among ions, eg. Cu- Zn, Cd- Zn, Cu-S-Mo, Fe- Zn, and Mn- Fe.
e. Chelation effects – positive or negative depending upon relative solubilities and dissociation constants.

General functions of minerals

Mineral nutrition is a complex one, since there are lot of interactions between the various minerals and some of them function in combination. However, a few general functions are given below.

a. *Electrochemical*: The elements are concerned in the maintenance of acid base balance, osmotic pressure and membrane permeability of cell in the body.

b. *Catalytic*: Nearly all essential elements are believed to have one or more catalytic functions in the cell as they are constituents of various enzymes and co- enzymes.

c. *Structural*: Large number of elements has a structural role in integrity of cell and the body as a whole. The frame work of the body (skeleton) and synthesis of structural protein are also dependant on so many minerals.

A number of elements have a unique functions e.g. calcium and phosphorus besides being a major constituent of bone and teeth are involved in wide range of metabolic reactions in gain of loss of energy and almost every energy form of energy exchange in the cell including the making and breaking of high energy phosphate bonds. It is also an integral part of protein molecules of the soft tissues of the body and of the nucleic acid and their derivatives that are involved in cell replication and transmission of the genetic code. Iron is the constituent of haem and play an important role in respiration. Co is a component of vitamin cyanocobalamin (B_{12}) and I is an constituent of thyroxine. Both the elements and vitamin are nevertheless concerned in a variety of metabolic processes. In ruminants including yak Co is necessary for the growth of certain bacteria which synthesizes vitamin B_{12} essential to the host animal. Though not much work has been conducted in yak as far as the minerals are concerned, and extensive work is required to conclude the function and requirement in yak.

5.3.6 Vitamins

Vitamins are usually defined as the organic compound which are required in small quantity compared to other nutrients for normal functioning and the physiological processes of body. The term vitamin is derived from 'vital amines' as it was thought that some food factors which contain amine nitrogen are essential for normal health. Later on it was known that certain vitamins contain amines. Many of the vitamins are not very stable and are destroyed by oxidation which is speeded up by certain metals, heat and light. These are the important things to be remembered during the formulation of ration and processing of feeds for animal. Most of the commercial companies are marketing the vitamins claiming to be stabilized. Though there are almost 15 vitamins known to be essential but not all of them are not dietary essential for farm animals as some of them are synthesized by the microbes in rumen and available to the host animals.

Classification

The vitamins are classified into fat soluble and water soluble vitamins on the basis of solubility in a particular solvent. Fat soluble vitamins are A, D_2, D_3, E and K whereas the water soluble vitamins are thiamin (B_1), riboflbin (B_2), niacin, pyridoxine (B_6), pantothenic acid, biotin, folic acid, chlorine, cyanocobalamin (B_{12}) and ascorbic acid or Vitamin C. Metabolic activity and deficiency symptom of fat and water soluble vitamins presented in table 5.3.

General functions of vitamins and deficiency symptoms

Name of the vitamin	Chemical name	Metabolic activity	Deficiency symptoms
Vitamin A	Retinol Retinal Retonoic acid	Oxidation- reduction cycle, visual cycle. Necessary for chondroitin sulphate. Maintenance of placenta in 2nd trimester	Dim light vision impaired. Rough skin (xerophthalmia) Reproductive failure
Vitamin D	Ergocalcipherol Cholecalcipherol	Absorption of Ca, P from gut. Necessary for calcification of bone matrix	Young animal- ricket Old animal- osteomalacia
Vitamin E	α Tocopherol*	Acts as antioxidant Normal phophorilation of ATP	Myopathy in calves Exudative diathesis
Vitamin K	Phylloquinone	Blood coagulation	Bleeding disease
Water soluble vitamins	Not required by the ruminants as these are synthesized in rumen and indirectly the requirement fulfils.		

* Vitamin E in yak milk is very high (2.74 mg/ml milk)as compared to Indian cow or Egyptian buffalo (Ahmad *et al.*, 2007)

5.4 Nutrient requirement of yak for various stages of life

Yak have intensive growth capacity and fattening potential in higher altitudes (Ghosh and Buragohain, 2004). Due to irrational stocking and rate and grazing pattern, unscientific feeding, imbalances in herbage supply both in quantity and quality especially during winter months, the calves or the adult yak suffer from poor growth, health problem and reduced fertility (Ghosh and Bandopadhyay, 2007). In addition, they reported that the supplementation of concentrate to the grazing dam reduces mortality of calves in the winter months. However, farmers rarely follow the scientific or balance feeding to the animals rather they fed their livestock depending on the availability of fodders. Reports are there that supplementation of concentrate significantly improved due to higher digestibility and intake of nutrients (Ghosh and Bandopadhyay, 2008).

5.4.1 Energy requirement for maintenance, growth and lactation

The energy requirement for maintenance is a useful term for expressing the level of the exogenous nutrient supply. It is defined as the metabolizable energy (ME) input per day at which the animals are in energy balance. Chinese workers used a respiration mask method to estimate the metabolizable energy requirement for maintenance (ME_m) in growing yak and found its value to be 460.2 kJ per kg $W^{0.75}$ per day and estimated the efficiency of utilization of metabolizable energy for maintenance (k_m) in growing yak is around 0.66. Though in India, not much work has been conducted and examined under field condition. As the yak is a grazing animal, two of its most common activities are standing up and moving on. Heat production to the difference in body size and breed, as smaller animals are expected to generate more heat during walking and these factors are to be remembered when ration is to be formulated for the animals.

Scientists have estimated metabolizable energy requirements for growth (ME_g) in growing yak through an energy balance trial by rationing their intakes of concentrate to a series of levels. The daily metabolizable energy requirement of growing yak was estimated as: ME (MJ/d) = $0.45W^{0.75}$ + (8.73 + 0.091 W) DG, where W is the body weight and DG is daily gain (kg), and the efficiency of utilization of metabolizable energy for growth (k_g) in yak is 0.49. Such a high value might be considered to apply only to diets rich in concentrates. However, similar results were obtained from other trials when animals were given coarse fodders.

Data on energy requirements for lactation are still scarce, as only preliminary studies on dietary energy digestion and metabolism in lactating yak have been conducted by few scientists. NRC on Yak, Dirang, Arunachal Pradesh has conducted few experiment under Indian context, but there is differences on requirement and farmers in Ladakh are least bothered about the energy requirement. They prefer to raise their animals only on fodders and hill grazing.

5.4.2 Protein requirement for maintenance, growth and lactation

Protein requirements for tissue maintenance, growth, lactation and wool and hair growth have been well discussed for many ruminants except the yak. There is as yet little information to define the protein requirement for maintenance in yak. Chinese workers used the comparative-slaughter method to measure the rumen degradable crude protein requirement for maintenance ($RDCP_m$) and obtained a value of $6.09W^{0.52}$ g per day for growing yak. For growing yak, the protein requirements include that for maintenance ($RDCP_m$) and for body weight gain ($RDCP_g$). According to Xue *et al.* (1994), the latter can be calculated as follows, $RDCP_g = (1.1548/DG + 0.509/W^{0.52})^{-1}$. Combining the value of $6.09W^{0.52}$ (for $RDCP_m$), the protein requirement of growing yak can be calculated as RDCP (g per day) = $6.09W^{0.52} + (1.16/DG+0.05/W^{0.52})^{-1}$, where DG is daily gain (g per day). However, these calculations need more experiments to validate them. For advanced pregnancy and lactating yak, as thumb rule in Ladakh, supplementation of wheat, buckwheat, barley or even rice @ 1-3 kg depending on body size is practiced. This indicates the requirement during the period is high but no organized study has been done or reported, hence, need to examine and conclude for the purpose. To date, little information on protein requirements for lactation is available. Only preliminary studies on protein digestion and metabolism in lactating yak have been conducted by some researchers.

5.5 Forage availability and pasture management

The uneven feed supply throughout a year suggests that grazing yak require feed supplements in the harsh winter on the Plateau. Harvesting oats and some productive perennials or imported crop residues (agricultural by-products) from nearby farming areas could be alternative feed sources to partly alleviate feed deficiency of yak in winter, provided this can be seen as cost-effective. Some feedstuffs and tree fodders have been evaluated by Mondal and Mir (2008) in

Ladakh and Ghosh and Konwar (2009) in North Eastern states for its chemical composition is shown in tables 5.4, 5.5 and 5.6.

As it is discussed, the yak rearing is primarily based on grazing on hills, pasture should be good enough to supply all the nutrients. They tend to graze on open meadows than in the forest cover and yak are able to access fodder from very steep slopes because of their foot characteristics. Pal (2003) reported in his study that on elevation of 4000-4300 m and in the summer about 25 species of plants were seen, out of which only 4 were grasses (*Carex* sp, *Cyperus* sp, *Festuca* sp) and rest were herbaceous. Plant density varied from 1742 to 3988 per sq m with the height varying from 9-10 cm. Unlike other ruminants, yak rarely browse shrubs, only during heavy snowfalls when hungry, they browse lightly on these plants. In some situation besides the shrub lands having species like *Dasiphora, Spiraea, Salix,Caragana* and *Rhodendron* offer valuable protein rich fodder supplement. The leaves or other edible part of available palatable fodder trees are valuable in supplementing green forage requirement as well as in the conserved form (Long, 1999). Pasture improvement is indeed a very tough task again in high altitude terrains. However, a well planned long term, inter-disciplinary holistic approach may be laid down to done the job. The populations of palatable species have dwindled considerably. The rehabilitation of these species along with other suitable pasture grass is of prime importance for pasture and grassland improvement and management in high altitudes. The natural grassland in sub-temperate, temperate and sub-alpine region are not fertilized in any form except the animal excreta and urine addition by the grazing animals. This leads to continuous depletion of natural plant and soil nutrients in the coming years resulting in poor growth of plant species. Singh (1995) observed that application of nitrogen @60 kg/ ha and phosphorus @ 30 kg/ ha will improve the herbage yield provided the pasture can be fertilized. Generally, uncontrolled and continuous grazing is prevalent in most of the pasture and grasslands perhaps due to rapid urbanization and population explosion. Although rotational system of grazing gives better result but not very easy task to adopt in hilly areas. The most desirable system of grazing would be that of periodic or deferred grazing by limiting number of livestock on the basis of carrying capacity of the grasslands. This system of grazing would give a better chance for self seeding and stand recovery.

Table 5.4 : Chemical composition of commonly used feeds, fodders and tree leaves under Kargil condition

Ingredients	OM	CP	EE	CF	NFE	NDF	ADF	Hemi-cellulose	Ash
Hay and tree leaves									
Alfalfa	90.28	18.12	2.29	25.31	34.31	40.99	30.77	10.22	9.72
Apple	90.82	10.41	2.12	19.65	48.72	60.29	26.39	33.90	9.18
Chenopodium	85.94	13.66	3.29	20.68	38.15	46.82	31.33	15.49	14.06
Buck wheat	89.53	13.76	2.11	23.64	38.27	40.41	28.06	12.35	10.47
Iris	91.47	17.68	3.35	23.51	34.29	53.62	30.82	22.80	8.53
Mulberry	88.48	20.74	2.52	21.72	33.37	31.34	19.31	12.09	11.52
Pea	91.07	20.19	2.69	16.84	40.81	38.38	27.8	10.58	8.93
Poplar	90.28	11.45	4.90	20.62	42.67	45.59	25.51	20.08	9.72
Red clover	90.76	15.08	1.59	23.64	39.76	42.95	24.13	18.82	9.24
Cicer	91.26	8.32	2.61	35.21	33.91	48.67	44.06	4.62	8.74
Sarsing	88.53	12.62	3.83	23.34	36.47	29.68	42.36	13.32	11.47
Plants with inferior grains									
Foxtail millet	91.52	12.62	3.40	28.65	35.10	80.25	41.28	38.97	8.48
Small millet	93.06	13.75	2.68	30.56	35.43	67.85	38.57	29.28	6.94
Buck wheat	92.62	12.49	8.57	24.61	35.95	28.62	16.12	12.50	7.38
Grains									
Oat	93.13	6.19	2.61	5.21	71.29	16.75	4.51	12.24	6.91
Wheat	93.35	8.12	2.39	6.33	65.76	15.25	5.73	9.52	6.51
Barley	95.38	7.05	2.51	4.61	70.03	15.36	4.61	10.75	4.31
Other feeds									
Wheat straw	90.42	3.32	0.8	43.75	32.05	83.53	55.84	27.69	9.58
Barley straw	91.85	2.28	1.12	47.72	29.93	78.39	53.15	25.24	8.15
Mustard siliqua	86.87	14.25	2.92	35.62	23.55	46.19	30.21	15.98	13.13

OM- Organic matter, CP- Crude protein, EE- Ether extract, CF- Crude fibre, NFE- Nitrogen free extract, NDF- Neutral detergent fibre, ADF- Acid detergent fibre (Mondal and Mir, 2008)

Table 5.5 : Chemical composition of tree fodders commonly fed to yaks of Arunachal Pradesh

Tree fodders	OM	CP	EE	NFE	NDF	ADF	Ash
Buddija astitica	90.4	14.0	0.7	78.8	58.9	41.1	6.6
Salyx humboltiana	89.1	14.5	2.3	72.3	56.6	29.8	11.9
Symplocus racemosa	91.9	11.0	1.9	79.0	46.5	38.4	8.1
Acer cambellii	94.5	15.1	1.5	77.9	45.6	28.5	5.6
Lingustrum myrsinites	95.3	9.8	1.4	84.1	47.8	36.6	4.7
Acer hookeri	94.6	7.1	2.0	85.5	36.4	23.1	5.4
Berberis sp	93.8	6.9	3.0	83.9	56.4	50.1	6.3
Quercus walliasehiana	94.1	18.4	5.0	70.7	75.5	54.8	5.9
Costanpsis sp	95.5	11.9	1.0	82.5	65.5	51.9	4.5

(Ghosh and Konwar, 2009)

Table 5.6 : Chemical composition of some tree fodders (DM basis) commonly fed to yak in Sikkim

Name	OM	CP	CF	EE	NFE	Ash
Artocarpus lakoocha	87.2	13.8	27.6	1.7	44.2	12.7
Ficus nemorlis	88.8	9.9	16.9	1.1	61.1	11.2
Premna mucronata	91.0	16.0	32.4	1.6	40.9	8.9
Ficus infectoria	91.1	14.9	49.8	2.7	23.8	8.8
Bohmeria macrophylla	85.0	16.5	36.8	1.4	30.3	14.9
Fecus bengalensis	88.9	11.9	40.6	2.1	34.2	11.2
Reevasia pubescens	85.2	19.4	44.6	2.6	18.7	14.7
Ficus hirta	83.2	16.8	21.6	1.2	43.5	16.6
Castopnopsis tribuloides	93.7	11.8	43.9	3.1	34.9	6.2
Bridelia retusa	89.5	12.0	24.0	1.0	51.3	10.5
Eurya japonica	93.9	9.7	17.4	4.9	62.0	6.0
Ampora wallichi	92.8	11.6	18.9	1.6	60.5	7.2
Exbucklandia populnea	92.1	6.8	20.2	1.7	63.4	7.8
Macranga nepalensis	95.0	16.8	14.7	2.9	60.6	5.0
Ficus elevate	85.7	17.7	28.2	1.0	38.7	14.3
Aldizia lebbek	83.4	14.7	40.7	0.7	37.2	6.6
Ficus elastica	89.9	7.4	30.0	2.5	49.9	10.1
Bauhinia purpurea	90.3	16.1	36.8	3.3	34.1	9.7

(Ghosh and Konwar, 2009)

References

Ahmad, F A, Bandopadhyay, S, Ghosh and M K Bhattacharya. 2007. Determination of alpha tocopherol in yak milk. *Indian Journal of Animal Sciences*. 77: 1048-49.

Blaxter, K L 1967. The energy metabolism of ruminants, 2nd Eds. Hutchinson & Co., London.

Ghosh M K and Konwar P. 2009.Yak husbandry and nutritional prospects in North East India. Proc. International conference on Yak husbandry-Challenges and Strategies held at National Research Centre on Yak, Dirang, Arunachal Pradesh India on 20-22 April, 2009. pp: 80-88.

Ghosh, M K and Bandopadhyay, S. 2007. Present nutritional status and future strategies for sustainable yak husbandry in India. *Indian Farming*. 56: 3-8.

Ghosh, M K and Bandopadhyay, S. 2008. Effect of feeding regimes on growth performance and nutrient digestibility of Indian yak under semi intensive system. *Indian Journal of Animal Sciences*. 78: 117-19.

Ghosh, M K and Buragohain, R. 2004. Feed Resources and nutritional status of yak. *Yak farming*. (Eds) Ramesha,K P and Sharma D K. pp- 49-60. NRC on yak, ICAR.Dirang, Arunalchal Pradesh.

Goering H K and Van Soest, P J.1970. *Forage fibre analyses*. USDA, Agriculture Handbook no- 379. Washington DC. USA.

Hino T and Kiroda, S.1993. Presence of lactate dehydrogenase and lactate racemase in Megasphora elsdenii grown on glucose of lactate. Applied Environmental Microbiology. 59: 255- 259.

Long, R J.1999. Nutritive value of natïve Tibetan forage. *Animal Feed Science and Technology*. 80: 101-113.

Maynard, L A, Loosli, J K, Hintz, H F and Warner, R G. 1979. *Animal Nutrition*. 7th Edition. TMH Edition. 136-85.

Mondal, G. and Kakati, B.K. 2008. Effect of feeding apricot oil cake on performance of key stone golden birds under cold arid condition. *Indian Journal of Animal Health*.47: 87-90.

Mondal, G. and M.S. Mir. 2008. Chemical composition of commonly used feeds and fodders available in Ladakh. *Indian Journal of Animal Sciences*. 78:328-330.

Mondal, G., Kakati, B. K. and Mehdi, M. 2011. Performance of broiler chicks under Kargil conditions. *Indian Journal of Animal Nutrition*. 28: 207-211.

Pal, R N. 2003. The yak husbandry in India. In: *The yaks* (Eds. G Weiner, H Jialin and L Ruijun).FAO, Regionl Office foe Asia and Pacific,Bangkok.pp-460.

Singh, V. 1995. Technology for forage production in hills of Kumaon. In: *New vistas in forage production* (Eds. C R Hazra and Bimal Misri).IGFRI, Jhansi. 197-202.

Visek, W. J. 1972. Effects of urea hydrolysis on cell lifespan and metabolism. Fed.Proc. 31: 1178-93.

□□□

Chapter 6

Management of Yak

Yak management characterises as a traditional trans-human system characterized by cyclical movements from low land to high lands to take advantage of seasonally available pastures at different elevation in the high altitude. It has remained traditional because of illiteracy, poverty, remoteness, a lack of political involvement and government services. Yak husbandry is an age-old practice and the only means of livelihood for many people living in high altitude areas from 3,000 m to 5,000 m. Managemental methods differ according to country and region, which is influenced by altitude, climate and topography. Culture and religion also plays a great role in yak management. As a unique animal inhabiting the very high mountain pastures, yak has no competition from any domestic livestock, but there is some competition from the wild animals. Yak has made life possible for man in one of the world's harshest environments. In purely pastoral areas, where cultivated agriculture is not possible, yak allow people to subsist and, in many areas, to live quite well (Miller, 1997). Domestic yaks are found grazing throughout the high elevation areas of the Hindu Kush and Karakoram in Afghanistan and Pakistan, the

Himalayas in India, Nepal and Bhutan, the Tibetan Plateau and Tian Shan Mountains of Northern China, Western and Northern Mongolia and also the adjoining areas of Russia and some of the Central Independent States of the former U.S.S.R. (Miller, 1996). Only a few mountainous countries have yak breeds. Their density ranges from 13 sq km/yak to 100 sq km/yak.

Management of yak ranges from the most primitive, apparently unchanged by the passage of time, to the technologically quite advanced practice. Yak farming systems are categorized into three systems namely nomadic, semi-settled and small-holder.

1. Since ancient times traditional **nomadic system** of yak rearing is practiced. Irrespective of the age and sex, the entire herds is kept together and allow grazing with sheep and horses. The yak raisers live with their animals and during the pasture growing season moved with them as necessitated by the availability of grazing and water.
2. In some areas, **semi-settled system** has been developed over the years. It develops from the early 1950s. As yak raisers settle in one place, they fence the pasture and supplements feeds during winter, such as oats, hay etc. They start agriculture operation where it is possible. In this system herd size are adjusted according to the availability of grazing land.
3. Since 1980, **small-holder farming** has been developed in China (Dong *et al.* 1999). Government lease the grazing land for about 50 years and area of grazing land is depending upon the family size.

Although yak is a member of the hoofed *bovidae* family, it is actually a unique species in itself. It differs from other bovines in several of its characteristics - for instance, its tail is similar to that of the horse but is less mobile, having long, thick wavy hair. Yak is a unique domesticated livestock species because of its ability to adapt to anoxic environment at high altitude, extreme cold conditions, high solar radiation, highly seasonal feed supply and grass shortages at higher altitudes. Yak can exploit pastures from 6,000 to 18,000 ft. They are well thrive with the low quality feed.

Yak also called as *chauri gua*, grunting cow, grunting ox, *sarlac, sarlik,* and *sarluc* etc. Yak is also known as 'camel of the snow'. Yaks are ox-like in build, with short, thick legs, humped shoulders, large up curved horns, and a thick coat that hangs down to the ankles. Wild yaks are scarcely found in isolated highlands at elevations above 14,000 ft (4,300 m) due to extensive hunting for meat and hide. Formerly they were found from Kashmir to west china. Yaks usually found in a group varies from 10-100. Males remain isolated, where as, old bulls lead females and younger animals. Domesticated yaks are smaller, with shorter horns than the wild yak.

6.1 Yak: Body conformation

The yak has a relatively large body size and short head with a wide forehead, and the clusters of hairs on the forehead are curled. Head is relatively heavy and bulky. Horn presents in both male and female yak, though those of the females are considerably smaller and shorter. The distance between the horns is large. Horns are very thick, grow out from the sides of the head and curve upwards. Horns grow up to 51 cm (20 inches) long in females, and 95 cm (38 inches) in males. Sometimes a few polled yaks are found (at the ration of 1:100) and not as greatly valued. The neck is short and wide, slightly higher than shoulder peak. The short slender neck is without dewlap. Small ears, deep chest, large belly but not sagging, straight and even back and waist, short legs are the other prominent features. The tail is broom-shaped. The hoofs are small and compact texture, with a narrow and sharp hoof tip, hard hoof edges and a close hoof fork. These hoof characteristics make deep imprints on the ground, and may be an adaptation to allow the yak to control its movement when going downhill. Thick hairs on the legs, belly and chest grow towards the ground. The average height of adult male yak is from 114.0 cm to 129.0 cm, and the body weight ranges from 220.1 kg to 348.7 kg. The average height of the adult female yak is from 103.6 cm to 112.8 cm and the bodyweight from 176.6 kg to 228.6 kg. Female yak matures at 3 years old and deliver the first calf at their 4 years of age. Generally, they deliver a calf every two years; the case of one calf one year is rare. The reproductive capacity reaches the highest from 6 to 12 years old and they stop breeding at age of 17 to 18 years. Yaks are very long-lived, with a life expectancy of 25 years (Lie, 2004).

The usual coat colour of yak is black with black nose (described as **imperial**) and with a grayish nose (described as **black**). Other predominant colours are black with some white markings on head, feet or tail (described as **trim**), which predominates, black and white piebald (described as **royal**) and a gold colour (described as **golden**), present in small numbers and said to be recessive to black. Grayish brown or pale yellow coats are not uncommon. Pure white yak are rare, but highly prized. The coat colour of the yak is genetically controlled.

Crossing of two trim yak can produce offspring that are black, trim, or royal in a ratio of 1: 2: 1 respectively (25% black, 50% trim, 25% royal) as shown in the Punnett Square below.

×	**Bb (Trim)**	
Bb (Trim)	BB (Black)	Bb (Trim)
	Bb (Trim)	Bb (Royal)

BB: homozygous dominant (black),
Bb: heterozygous (trim),
bb: homozygous recessive (royal)

Golden yaks are the result of a cross between two black yaks that both contain the rare golden yak gene. Crossing golden yak parents can also produce golden offspring.

All category of yak attain peak weight and body condition annually towards the end of the warm season in September and October and are in their poorest conditions in March and April at the end of the dry harsh winters. Lack of adequate care and feeds during winter are reportedly as the main reasons for the poor growth rate and condition of animals. Body weight of yak cows ranges from 285-330 kg, while yak bulls are slightly heavier than female and body weight varies from 400-550 kg. Young bulls (about 3-4 years old) used for meat purpose and their body weight varies 320-350 kg under satisfactory conditions of maintenance and feeding. Full size is achieved in six to eight years.

Yak grunt when agitated, hungry, or calling their young. Otherwise, they make no sound at all. Yaks are inquisitive, intelligent, and quiet animals each with their own distinct personality. They learn to come when called and have a highly developed sense of sight and hearing.

6.2 Acclimatization at the high altitude

Yak posses valuable unique characteristics which help it's keeping and breeding at severe extreme cold condition. They can easily withstand average annual temperature of -8°C and winter temperature of –40°C. these unusual characteristics are due to its long and dense hair coat, very thick hide, large thoracic cavity, respiratory exchange potential higher than in cattle (large alveolar area; larger, more numerous erythrocytes with higher haemoglobin content) and sizable amount of subcutaneous fat. Sweat glands are less developed in yak and the subcutaneous fat is more developed than other related animals. The skin has few wrinkles and the surface area of the yak is relatively small per unit bodyweight (0.016 m^2/kg). Its neck, the outer side of its legs, and its flanks, are covered with long, flowing, fine hair. These physical advantages hamper exchange of heat exchange and preserve energy, which is very much essential to this extreme environment. Another extraordinary characteristic of yak is that they can tolerate very low oxygen tension at very high altitude and therefore, resistant to hypoxic condition. Because of its large heart, lungs and a high erythrocyte count, the yak can tolerate the low oxygen content in the air of high altitude. Short neck, narrow muzzle and mobile lips help them to graze the more nourishing low-growing vegetation which cattle and other domestic animals cannot graze. Yak have unique ability to scoop out the snow for feeding during the winter, and less weight loss during winter compared to cattle and sheep on the same pastures (Bonnemaire 1984). The forelegs are short but as thick and strong as the hindlegs. Yak is a sure-footed climber. Strong legs and hoof structure helps them to walk smoothly in the steep rocky slopes. In extreme winter, although severe scarcity of vegetation at high altitude deserts, still yak can get their feed until the snow is soft and not deeper than 10-12 cm. These qualities of yak help to adapt well to the severe conditions of their habitat and to reproduce at low temperatures.

6.3 Management of Animal

Management of yak ranges from the most primitive, seemingly unchanged by the passage of time, to the technologically quite advanced practice.

6.3.1 Calf rearing

One of the most critical times in the life of an animal is shortly after birth. Due to the seasonal breeding pattern of the female yak, most calves are born from April to July, with May the peak month. Around 60 percent of yak calves born in between the end of April and beginning of May. Parturition takes place as effortless, problem free, and finished within very short time. Almost all births take place during the day and only very few occur at night when the yak cows are normally at the yak raisers' campsite. Naval cord is broken automatically by the act of mechanical stretching when its mother stands up after delivery or by the yak calf falling down. Although the broken cord is not sterilized, inflammation as well as infections is rare. Special attention should be given to the newborn yak calf. The dam generally licks the newborn calf for about ten minutes, after which the calf attempts to stand up and suck (after about 20 - 30 minutes) and then starts running. They can survive temperatures as low as -30°C. The preferred temperature for well-nourished yaks is about 10°C but increases to above 18°C if they are malnourished. Yak calves suck their dam. If dam of the calf dies, then only artificial rearing is practiced with the foster mother. Fostering is only attempted when another cow lost her calf at the same time. Because of her strong maternal instinct, a yak cow that has lost her calf can be persuaded to accept another calf that needs to be fostered. This can be done either by smearing her milk or salt on the calf that will stimulate the foster dam to smell and lick the new calf and adopt it as her own, or put the hide of her dead calf on the intended fosterling. Like calf of the cow, yak calf also receives colostrum for the first two days and the quality of the colostrum is better than the milk produced thereafter (Table-6.1). The calf sleeps a lot the first day. First one month all milk is allowed to calves. At about seven to ten days old yak calves start nibbling the grass, but they have not been observed to ruminate before the age of 12 days. At the age of one month, when dam starts to be milked, yak calves continue to suck and graze beside its dam. At night the calf is separated from the dam. The calves are then penned or tethered to long ropes near the herders' tent or hut to protect them from predators. If calf become ill or her mother produces too little milk then only calves are allowed to stay with her mother at night. This process continues until the cold season starts. In extreme winter months the calf and her mother allowed to stay together all day and the calf usually obtain little amount of milk through suckling. At this time yak cows are not milked.

Table 6.1 : Composition colostrum and normal milk in yak (Zhang Rongchang, 1989 and Liu Haibo, 1989)

Milk type	Milk solid (%)	Fat (%)	Protein (%)	Lactose (%)	Ash (%)	Density kg/litre
Colostrum	32.0 - 34.5	13.2 - 15.8	15.1 - 17.1	1.7 - 1.9	0.9 - 1.1	1.03 - 1.07
Normal milk	16.9 - 17.7	5.5 - 7.2	4.9 - 5.3	4.5 - 5.0	0.8 - 0.9	1.03 - 1.04

6.3.1.1 Availability of milk to the yak calf

As milk production of the yak is very low. Whatever they produce that is sufficient for the survival of their calf. When yak females are milked definitely it affects the growth of the calves. Calf's growth depends upon at what extend the milking is done by the yak raiser. Availability of milk to the yak calf depends upon the frequency of milking and amount of milk allowed. This practiced are classified into three category, 1) to give the calf exclusive access to the milk of its dam (the dam is not milked), 2) to milk the dam once a day and allow the calf the remainder, and 3) to milk the dam twice a day and allow the calf what remains.

6.3.1.2 Weaning

Weaning involves removing of young one from its mother and terminate suckling. Although yak cow has strong maternal instinct, weaning of calves is accepted. At the time of weaning they only produce simple grunts, no bellowing or mooing. Neither dam nor calf shows any type of stress due to weaning. Calf is weaned at the age of six to twelve months provided her mother become pregnant. If the dam is not pregnant then calf usually stays with their dam through a second summer. In majority cases yak cow does not conceive in the same year of calving. For successful weaning calf is separated from the dam and placed into another herd. In condition, farmer has single herd and calf still try to suckle her mother, then a piece of wood (both ends pointed) about 20 cm long is placed through the nasal septum between the nostrils. Wood is only removed when the calf stops the attempt at suckling. At the time of weaning their body weight ranges from 65-70 kg. After weaning the young animals are incorporated into the mixed herd.

6.3.1.3 Neonatal Growth

Newborn yaks are smaller than cattle calves. Birth weight of calves varies between 9 to 20 kg, which is about 5.9 percent of dam's weight, whereas in cattle, calves birth weight varies from 6.5 to 8 percent of the live weight of adults. The relatively low birth weight is a consequence of a relatively short gestation length (average 258 days) and that the fact that in mid- and late pregnancy the yak, typically, has to exist on ground that is frozen and covered with ice and snow. Also, the yak does not normally have the benefit of supplementary feeding. The growth rate of the calves is fast in the first few months. Their survival rate in coming winter depends upon the calf's initial growth. Therefore, calves have born early in the summer season gain more body weight before reaching to the winter and subsequently better chance of survival. Males become heavier than females, but they grow relatively more slowly in the early years of life and continue to grow for longer. Malnutrition appears to be the main cause of slow growth. Growth rate of the calves depends on the access of the whole amount of dam's milk. The average live weight (kg) of yaks at the age of 1 month 21-22, 3 months 33-35, 6 months 57-60, 9 months 140-145, 12 months 150-160 and 16 months 175-180 kg (Sarbagishev *et al.*, 1989). Calf energy intake comes from milk and forage. Body weight of calves showed a rapid growth up to 2.5 years old and then a flat curve until four years old, when the animals are strong enough to seek out better pastures. This is probably due to natural selection resulting in the survival of the strongest one. From four years of age body weight varied with seasons. Calves are exceptionally disease-resistant and cold hardy due to their wool coat. Scours are extremely rare, and only occur in extremely wet and muddy conditions. All the calves loose their body weight during winter and spring season and, regain its lost body weight and also additional growth occur in the next summer season. In the first year 12 percent body weight loss takes place of yak calf's in the winter and spring season, where as in the succeeding winter and spring the body weight loss at the tune of 25 percent.

6.3.1.4 Tethering of calves

Normally, the calves are tethered when their dams are milked. When the dam is milked only once daily, the calf is tethered and kept from the dam for a relatively short time only and grazes and drinks water alongside the dam for most of the day. Calves with dams milked twice a day are tethered for much of the day and have perhaps only four to five hours of time during which they move around at pasture with their dams. After peak lactation, the calves are allowed to graze with their mothers during the whole day.

6.3.1.5 Protection

Yak cows are attentive mothers. Due to very strong maternal instinct yak dams are remarkably protective of their own calves, as well as other calves in the herd, from any perceived threat including dogs and other predators. If any intruder enters their safe-space they will give a series of grunt-snort warnings combined with head shakes before further protective measures are taken. Dam usually protects calves from anything intent to causing harm.

6.3.1.6 Dehorning

Dehorning usually not done by the yak raiser. If dehorned, then it is done at the very early age by using dehorning paste. Dehorning is advantageous for the trainer/handler's safety. However, the yak will be at a disadvantage state for defense with other yaks.

6.3.1.7 Castration

Castration is the removal of testicles of bull. Castration is a common practice among the yak raiser. Other than breeding bull, all the young males are castrated. Castration is usually done at the age of 3-4 years with the traditional method. Young male yak is tied up and grounded on its side. The lower part of the scrotum is then sliced open and the testicles pushed out. The cords are crushed. The open wound then sterilized with boiling mustard or iodine solution. Most of the herders conduct castration. Castrated animals are maintained for meat purpose.

6.3.1.8 Identification

Identification of animals is a requirement in the management of individual animal as well as herd. Usually yaks are identified by the colour and body confirmation by the yak raiser. However, ear tag is applied in some advanced yak raiser.

6.3.1.9 Calfhood diseases

Owing to their strong adaptability in the harsh environment, the calfhood diseases are very limited. They seldom suffer to the diseases. However, particularly calves in their early age may suffer to calf scours. Gid diseases (*Multiceps multiceps*) is not uncommon in some areas and which causes high calf mortality rate.

Calf scours

Calf scours mostly occur from birth to four days of age. Particularly the spring-born calves are most susceptible. In some studies it has been reported that calf scours in early age is the major cause (about 20-30 percent) of calf mortality and causative organism is *E. coli* (Lensch, 1996). Infected calves develop profuse diarrhoea, white mucous stools are of a thin, pasty to watery consistency, sometimes containing blood. Calves are treated with a drink made from medicinal herbs as veterinary care is least available to the yak raiser. Where limited facility is available, recovery rates are high with the treatment with anti-bacterial drug. However such treatment is not widespread.

6.3.1.10 Calf Mortality

Lack of proper care and undesirable milking of dam are the major cause of calf mortality. When dams are not milked and the calves are allowed to suckle, the survival rate increases. Survival rate sharply decline if the dams are milked. A new born calf survival rate is also greatly depends upon the maintenance of body temperature at the 2-3 hours of life. In the first hour of life, calves body temperature fall (0.38°C), and returned to normal, after three hours. Fall of body temperature is correlated with the birth weight of calves (the greater the weight, the less the temperature loss). Excessive fall of body temperature may cause death of the new born calf. Ambient temperature also plays significant role in the initial fall of body temperature. Sicknesses of calves are mostly related to the poor nutrition. Other causes are from predation by wild animals and accidental falls to the ditch.

6.3.2 Rearing of heifer

Heifer is the future replacement stock of the herd. Growth of yak depends upon the availability of milk at the calfhood. Weaker yak calf leads to the development of weak and underweight heifer, because of the cyclicity of the body weight change. Yak is slow maturing animal its growth largely depends on the biomass and grass nutrients of the pasture, changing among seasons. Better-grown heifer produces more milk. During cold weather, yaks must increase their metabolism to maintain body temperature. If the intake of natural forage does not meet their nutritional needs, they will use stored reserves, thereby decreasing weight and body condition. Lack of adequate care and fodders during winter are reportedly as the main reasons for the poor growth rate and condition of these animals. Yak gain weight during the warm season from June to October and loose weight during the cold season from November to following May. The ratio of body weight gain to loss decreases with increasing age until body maturity (at about 7 years of age for males and 5 years for females) and the ratio tend to be about one. Hence, the growth pattern of the yak consists of peaks (the heaviest weights) and valleys (the lightest weights) occurring every year. Growth rate is much faster between 2 and 4 years of age when the animals are strong enough to seek out better pastures. This is probably due to natural selection resulting in the survival of the strongest of the lot. Peak size in males is attained around 5 years of age and in females at around 4.

Yak heifers reach puberty at the age of 16 to 40 months, depending upon the managemental condition. Age of puberty of yak heifer depends on whether their mothers were also being milked while suckling. If dams are milked and calf does not get sufficient milk, then heifer reaches puberty at a later age. When dams are not milked, calves get whole amount of milk and therefore heifer reaches puberty earlier, mostly at the age of 16-18 months. The heifers usually calve for the first time at the age of three years. In rare cases heifers may come in heat at the age of 8-10 months but no fertilization has been observed at this age. Yak heifers conceive at two years of age and calve at three years of age. At first calving the live weight of yak cows should be not less than 255 kg.

6.3.3 Rearing of pregnant animals

Yaks are seasonally polyoestrous. Mating begins in late June. Sometimes it begins in early June. Mating continues till late October, in rare cases till December or January. Barren female attain heat in June-July while depending on the time of calving, recently calved yak attain heat from July till September. Conception rate is very high in female yak. They graze through out the year. Due to the low availability pasture grass and poor of pasture quality, nutritional deficiency is very common among the pregnant yak. Therefore, the physical condition at its lowest in mid and late pregnancy, although requirement is higher for the foetal growth at this stage. Body condition of the dam at the time of pregnancy plays a great role in the survival of calves. Calves birth weight highly dependent on the nutrient availability of the dam during pregnancy. Birth weight of the calves directly related to the initial fall of body temperature (average fall 0.38°C), as birth weight is higher the less is the body temperature loss. Too much fall of body temperature may cause death of the new born calf. At first calving, the live weight of yak cows should be not less than 255 kg, at the second and subsequent calving 295 kg. Nutritional deficiency usually results in low birth weight of calves and difficult labour is rare because of the small size of the calf. In rare case if assistance is required, then it is very difficult to deliver it as pregnant yaks are hard to approach during delivery because of their highly protective maternal instinct. However, assistance is necessary when a yak cow gives birth to an F1 (interspecies hybrid) calf, because sires of large exotic breeds were used to produce the hybrid. When calving is assisted, the navel cord is cut by knife; otherwise it is broken after delivery when yak female stands up. Broken naval cord is not usually sterilized as infection is very rare. Pregnant yaks may abort or even die during very cold weather. Therefore they should be protected when the environmental temperature is too low.

6.3.4 Rearing of lactating animals

Although yaks are multipurpose animals, they are raised mainly for milk production. Yaks give birth to single calves in alternate years, but in areas of poor grazing, a few may give birth only once every three years. In this traditional system, yaks are grazed all the year round without supplementation during winter.

The milking process is started one month after parturition. Even in the extreme winter the female yaks can produce milk, but the yak raiser do not milk them in order to keep them and their calves healthy. In the very next year summer season (i.e., second year of calving), the female yak again starts giving milk, provided the yak female do not conceive. Their milk yield is about $\frac{1}{2}$ or $\frac{1}{3}$rd to that in the first year of calving and also peak milk production in the month of July and August. These females are called "half-lactation cows" by local people. This is a unique lactation phenomenon among yak. On the other hand, lactating yaks in the year of calving are normally called "full-lactation cows. Yak does not dry off when milking ceases at the end of the warm season, and the calf, when present, continues to take some milk. The mammary gland of half-lactating yaks maintained an active secreting state, although it has undergone a longer period of lactation than yaks at late lactation. The reduced milk yield in the half lactating yaks might be caused by the normal involution of mammary gland, similar to cows prior to entering the dry period; as a result of endocrine changes. Oestradiol-17b is an important hormone for the development of mammary gland and level of oestradiol-17b is low in half-lactating yaks which might be responsible for the reduced lactation yield (Yu-cai *et al.*, 2002).

6.3.4.1 Milking

6.3.4.1.1 Milking Site

Three different sites of milking are usually observed in different parts of yak raising areas.

- Yak female is tethered at the campsite for milking. From the calfhood yak is accustomed with the tethering practice. Calf is either tethered or kept inside corral. Calves are placed around the dams, so that it can see it's calf during milking. Tethering is done by tying a neck rope by a wooden peg to a long rope with many rings. The rope is fixed to the ground at the campsite. Yak remembers the position and rope of tethering within a short span. If they are shifted from one campsite to other site, then also they accustom with it very quickly.
- Milking within the stall is practiced in some areas. At the time of milking milkers call the yak by using charming, eloquent names given at the time of first milking. The milking stall is having wall in the left and front side (100 - 120 cm long, 60 - 80 cm wide and 60 - 80 cm high) and other two sides open. Walls and floor made up on stone slabs and one wooden pole is placed inside the stall to secure the animal. another type
- In some areas, milking takes place anywhere on the campsite without tethering at all. Milker approach to the yak cow with bucket in one hand and calf in tow.

6.3.4.1.2 Milking process

Yak milk and its products are mostly consumed by local people. Yak raisers have developed their own milking skills through a long history of yak keeping. All of these traditional skills and technologies have their own characteristics. Only hand milking is practiced. Milking is done at the campsite. Size of udder as well as teat is smaller than cattle. Udder is covered with hair. Udder washing is usually done before milking. Order of milking is fixed and which is according to the tethering arrangement of the calves. Let down process is nearly impossible without stimulation from the calf. Calf is released just before milking. Then, calf runs to its mother and starts suckling. After about half to one minute (let down time), it is held back and tethered, kept in corral or held by children or older person within sight of the cow. A knot is sometimes applied to the hind legs by using a short rope. Milker remains silent and sits on the right side during milking. Milking pail hung from a hook on a girdle. Butter spreads on the side of the pail, to lubricate the teats. The teats are squeezed quite hard in between fingers (about 80 squeezes per minute). Milking process is laborious because of the strong sphincter muscles in small teats (2.5-4 cm). To keep calm and quite at the time of milking, the yak cow generally offers a small amount of barley powder (about 250 g) mixed with salt. Residual milk is accounted for about 13 percent, but this is normally left by the yak raises for the calf. It is better not to changed milker very often as yak are very sensitive to smells and voices.

For milking in summer, yaks are rounded up every evening. After evening milking, yaks are freed and allowed them to graze during the night until dawn. In the morning they are again rounded up for milking. Young calves are either penned or tethered to a long rope at night to prevent suckling their. After milking in the morning, they are usually driven in a different part of the pasture so that the milk is saved for the evening.

6.3.4.1.3 Milk yield

Genetically yak is low milk producer. The amount of milk they produce is sufficient for the well development of their calves. Adult yak females produce between 200 and 400 litres of milk in the year of calving, and when combined with that used for their young, about 700 kg and about two thirds of that amount in the second year without calving again. Daily milk yield of yak cow ranges from 1 to 2.5 kg. Milk yield of the female yak depends upon several factors.

- *Age and Parity*: Like cow milk yield also varies according to the parity in yak female. First calved heifer can produce milk as high as 54 percent of that of adult yak female. The milk production slowly increases upto 9 years old, after which milk production begins to decline and dramatically drops after 13 years old.
- *Weather* : In the summer season, variable temperature affects the milk yield. Yak produces less milk at too high temperature with strong solar radiation and a lack of wind on clear days. However, it can produce more milk within short periods of cloudy or rainy time. On a cloudy day and rainy day 1.9 percent and 7.7 percent

percent, respectively, higher milk production recored in comparison to a clear day (Xu Guilin *et al.*, 1983). It has been suggested that high environmental temperature might prevent yak female from producing heat, thus the milk yield dropped with the decreased metabolism. Conversely, low environmental temperature might cool down the yak female, so the milk yield goes up with the increased metabolism. Precipitation can also influence milk yield to some extent. Decreased temperature caused by raining might be the main contributor to the increased milk yield. The optimum temperature for yak is around 5-13°C. In harsh winter, female yaks can give milk (about 100g/day), but the yak raisers do not milk them in order to keep mother and their calves healthy.

- *Availability of pasture grass*: Milk production is highly variable according to the availability of pasture grass (quantity, growth status and nutritive value of the herbage). In month of June to August there are plenty of good quality green grasses, therefore milk yield increases upto 22-25 percent compare to previous months. These months are known in yak-producing areas of China as the "golden age". In September and October, as air temperature falls, the nutritive value declines as the grass produces seeds and then wilts, and the crude fibre content is high, consequently milk yield starts decline. In winter animals hardly find any grass and milk production further decline and finally stopped. this state continue upto spring season

- *Milking frequency in a day*: Like cow total milk yield strongly correlated with the number of milking a day. Because of the fact that udder of the yak is too small; hence it can not accumulate much milk in its udder. Yak female gives about one third more milk, in total, if stimulated by milking twice daily compared with once-a day milking (Cai and Wiener, 1995). However, too much milking is undesirable, because it affect negatively the growth of calves. Milking three times a day is also practiced in yak female that do not have a calf at foot.

- *Time of calving*: Time of calving is another important factor for the total milk production. Those female yak calved early on the summer season i.e., calved in March or April can produced upto 360kg of milk as compared to a Yak that calved in June, producing a mere 150kg. It is due to early calved female yak is having more lactation length compare to late calver.

- *Peak milk yield*: Unlike cattle, yak female does not have lactation peak in relation to the date of calving. Peak milk yield is solely dependent on the availability of the pasture grasses. Highest milk production is usually recorded in July and August month irrespective of age, parity and breed type when grass is abundant and nutritious, then declines as the grass dries off gradually before or in October and milk production decline slowly.
- *Milker's skill*: Skillfulness or/and milking speed of milkman also influence milk yield.
- *Supplementary feeding*: As yak rearing system is based on the grazing. Generally no supplementary feeding is allowed to them. The milk yield varies considerably with the supplementary feeding. Oat hay, barley straw etc., are supplemented to female yak. Milk production increases with the supplemented diet, but the lactation length does not change (Zhou, 1984). Fat content of the milk decreases due to increase milk yield, however total fat content of the milk increases.
- *Feeding of additive*: Imbalance of minerals is prominent and it limits the production of yak milk. Supplementation of salt-lick block resulted in 15.5 percent and 14.8 percent increase of milk yield in full lactating yak (milking in the year of calving) and half lactating yak (milking in second season without calving again), respectively (Yuan Youqing, 1994). Protein deficiency is another limiting factor. Protein supplementation in the form of UMMB (urea molasses mineral block) contained 10 percent urea, 0.1 percent mixed minerals and trace elements (Fe, Zn, Mg, Cu, etc.) in summer significantly improve milk production. As natural source many species of shrubs' leaf (contain 25-35 percent protein) are ideal protein supplements for grazing yak (Dong Shikui *et al.*, 2002). Remoteness of the yak rearing area is the major bottle neck for the supplementation. It not only increases the costs of supplying supplements (if not locally available) but also there may not be a ready market for extra produce. Usually ill health and poor production are the criteria for the supplementation. Many yak dies due to extreme climate and supplements (feed block, salt lick etc) may act as insurance against it.

6.3.4.1.4 Milk composition

Yak milk is a highly energizing food. Yak milk is less familiar with due to its remote geographical location. Detail chemical composition of yak milk is described in the table-6.2. Milk solid (dry matter) varies around 15-18 percent. Composition of the yak and its hybrids milk is far higher than cattle and very close to buffalo (Zhang Rongchang, 1989). Like milk yield, composition of yak milk greatly varies with climate change and grass availability and their chemical composition in their pasture. Milk solids, lactose, protein and amino acids in yak milk are at their highest in mid-lactation and fat percentage increases continuously as the lactation progresses. Milk fat increases with the progress of lactation as milk yield starts decline after July. Milk fat percentage go as high as 14 percent in the cold season when daily milk production as low as 100 g per day. Milk protein and lactose increase at the early lactation, peak at the mid lactation and drop at the late lactation. Fat content in yak milk is negatively correlated to the milk yield (Cai, 1989; Zhang, 1989). Average diameter of the milk fat globules (μ) is 4.39. Due to the large size of fat globules, the loss of butter during separation is lower, and 97 percent of butter is extracted. The proportion of essential to nonessential amino acids is 0.8:1 (Zhang Rongchang *et al.*, 1986). About 22 kinds of fatty acids are found in the yak milk. The saturated and unsaturated fatty acids constitute 65.2 percent and 34.8 percent, respectively, of the total fatty acids in the yak milk. Low molecular weight fatty, capryne, caprice and caprylic acids, which are responsible for the smell and taste of fat, they constitute 7.2 percent of the total fatty acids. Among the saturated acids, palmitic (29.2%) and stearic (14.9%) are dominant. Yak milk is rich in carotene; the butter is of yellowish colour and very delicious (Indra and Magash, 2000). Half-lactation yaks have higher contents of protein and fat, and activities of g-GT (Glutamyl transpeptidase) and AKP (Alkaline phosphatase) in milk than full lactation yaks. Half-lactation yaks resemble yaks in a late stage of lactation in their biochemical composition of milk (Zheng, 1994).

Table 6.2 : Composition of Yak Milk

Specific gravity	**1.037-1.038**
Fat (%)	5.8-6.3
Protein (%)	4.80-5.75
Casein (%)	3.8
Lactose (%)	5.32-5.66
Ash (%)	0.86-0.93
Total solids (%)	16.84-17.35
Calcium ppm (mg/kg)	12880
Iron ppm (mg/kg)	3.90
Potassium ppm (mg/kg)	8592
Magnesium ppm (mg/kg)	904
Phosphorus ppm (mg/kg)	8517
Zinc ppm (mg/kg)	46
Copper ppm (mg/kg)	0.35
Manganese ppm (mg/kg)	1.0
Selenium ppm (mg/kg)	0.18

6.3.5 Management of male yak

Male yaks are economically important as the female ones. Other than breeding they also play significant role by providing transport and draught power. They are also a standing insurance against bad times as they could be easily sold in times of need and fetch good prices. Yak steers (generally castrated around 4 years of age) are used for plowing and for threshing grain. The young yaks are trained to carry loads and plough fields. A wooden ring is fixed at the nose by piercing the nose. This ring secured with a rope to control easily. While training them as pack yaks, they are secured by ropes to a dominant yak, and to plough, they are paired up with stronger and dominant yaks. The training process to carry loads and plough in the field is started when they are young one. Yak carries about 60 kg of load, loaded in equal halves on either flank of their back upon a saddle. Yak ploughs more efficiently than cattle. A pair of yak ploughs as much as 3 times the area ploughed by a pair of bullocks in a day.

Depending upon the rearing condition of male yaks the age of puberty varies. If their mothers were milked when they were suckling they mostly reach puberty at the age of 2 years and if their mothers get better feed in the suckling period, at the age of 15-18 months. At 3 years of age, the yak bulls consider for breeding. Bulls at the age of 1.5-3 years should have a live weight of 340-420 kg, at the age of 4-5 years 480 kg or more. Average weight of adult Yak bull is 550 - 680 kg, although one yak bull in Canada was reported to weigh 820 kg.

Bulls selected for breeding purpose are either from own herd or purchased. Following are the selection criteria for breeding yak bulls

Body size:	The breeding bull should be bigger than other bulls of the same age
Body conformation:	It should have a proportionate body and not posses any deformity
Colour:	Black with white tail and spot on the face is the most preferred colour
Horns:	The horns should be large and symmetric as they are highly correlated with the fighting ability of the bull
Temperament:	The bull should be dominating and aggressive to be able to fend of challengers

Male yaks graze freely among the different herds of females day and night and rounded up only when administering salt or for other purposes, therefore, bear almost no cost of rearing. Male pedigree of the progenies remains unknown, apart from judgment of phonological features because males are mated freely. Cares are taken to prevent predation by the wild animals. Breeding males are left open for free grazing on communal pasture land. They spend most of the year either alone or in groups of up to twelve. During the mating season, which begins in September, the bulls join the herd and fight other bulls for the females. Some amount of Mustard oil and oil cakes offers to the breeding bull at the end of the mating season. Yak bulls are not shorn of hair or combed of its wool, which help to enhance its size. Usually, the productive life of a breeding bull is up to 12 years of age after which it becomes incapable of defending its status and is castrated or culled.

6.4 Routine farm management

Yak has strong adaptability at the high altitude where other animal can not thrive. Harsh climatic condition prevents higher productivity level of this species. Availability of the feed and fodder resources are very limited and season oriented. They require minimum mangemental intervention, as they are very much hardy animal. They hardly demand any type of supplementation. However, supplementation improves their productivity level significantly. Within the limited resources yak raiser routinely follow some techniques/methods for the higher productivity as well as welfare of the yak.

6.4.1 Herd management

Several small holder combined their herd and driven to the common summer pasture. Allotment of pasture depends on the milking regime of the animals. The division of herd is applied primarily to daytime grazing in the warm season. At night, the yak tended to be divided again by family ownership and the different types of yak mixed and kept near the family tent. In the early summer they are brought to progressively higher pastures. During the monsoon (June to September), the herds reach the highest alpine pastures. Families living in a transportable shelter. They drive the animal from one pasture to another. They remain in one area for about two weeks. This practice continues until winter. All the animals brought back to the village in the early winter. During the cold season, the families collect back their own yak to keep them on winter-spring pastures, which nowadays are increasingly fenced. If supplement feeds are available, then in winter and spring they are supplemented with turnips, crop residues, leaf fodder, hay and small amounts of maize flour. Adult animals remain in the nearby grazing field. The level of supplementary feeding is very low and inadequate to meet the nutrient requirements of animals in winter.

When the herd size is large then they are divided into two or more sub-herds. Females and young calves are separated from the pack and growing male stock. Milking and dry females again divided into two different groups. Milking females and young calves are allotted the best and most accessible pastures. The dry female, young bulls and heifers occupy marginal pastures away from the main campsites. However, the pack animals are driven to the uppermost reaches of the ridge for the whole summer rounding up only when required. In summer, between July and August, the calves are driven in a separate direction from the dams so that they do not suckle the milk during the day.

6.4.2 Controlling the herd

Temperamentally, yak are at varying times wild or timid, cowardly and yet aggressive. Yak has strong herding instinct. From the calfhood yak are trained in such a way that one person control and manage a large herd. Yak raisers train yak to obey commands both by voice and by use of small stones that are either thrown or projected with a sling. The yak raisers usually stay with the yak herd to protect them from predators especially at the times of calving, and to prevent the herd from straying onto another's territory which is set aside for other herds. As yak are timid in nature, the yak raiser cannot follow too closely behind the herd for fear of it scattering. For controlling the herd the person has to select a high spot of the ground and observe the herd.

The yak raiser produce special sounds to call the yak and throw a small stones to give signal to return to the herd. A sling is generally used to through the stones. Yak hair, down hair (fine hair) or sheep's wool is used to weave the sling. Length of the sling varies from 100 - 120 cm. It has an elliptical net at its centre (7 x 15 cm) to hold the stone. One skilled person can project a stone more than 100 m with use of sling. Sound produced from the stone flying through the air at great speed and the sound of the sling (like the crack of a whip) gives an alarm signal to the yak. Depending upon the direction of the sound yak understand which way to go and whether to advance, gather or disperse.

6.4.3 Tethering

Tethering is a process where a rope or chain is used for tying an animal to a fence, post, etc., so that it cannot move away from a particular place. The animals are tethered near the campsite to protect them from predators and for purposes of milking the females. Normally, the tethering site is square and enclosed by several layers (circles) of the rope with the wooden bars at the corners. Once yak return from the pasture after grazing, at night they find their respective places (which is fixed for a particular yak) at the tethering site. The rope used for tethering the animals is usually made up of yak hair or skin. The length of the rope varies according to the type of animals. Pack yak require larger rope (50-60 cm) in comparison to the female and calves (40-50 cm). The gap between two yak usually 2 m and gap between two stretches of rope is usually 5 m. Regarding arrangement of the animals at the tethering site, strong, aggressive pack steer and first calved female are placed to the most outside row which is farthest from the yak raisers tent. Next inner rows are allotted for adult female, two years old calves and one year old calves, respectively. Milking females are placed near the calves.

6.4.4 Housing

Yak is found at the highest elevations where intrinsic adaptation to the harsh environment is of paramount importance. As a whole, yak are regarded as reasonably tame and, with few exceptions, easily handled and easily confined by fencing a simple four strand barbed wire fence is all that is required. It is common practices that yak are kept out-of-doors the year round. Provision of housing even in winter could not generate huge success. Therefore, they do not demand elaborate housing facilities.

In summer, unusual temperature rise leads to panting like a dog due to less developed sweat gland in yak. They wade into streams and ponds, catching a breeze, laying in the shade of trees or lying in a low spot where the earth is cooler due to excess heat in summer. Yak does not like close housing facilities like other livestock species to get rid from the scorching summer. Even in winter, they prefer to use shade shelters with open sides, or the shelter of trees. They prefer to eat snow rather than drink water. They can mix very well with other livestock. Existing cattle facilities can easily be used. Any fence that holds in cattle will work just as well for Yaks.

Housing in terms of pen is provided to yak female in their late pregnancy and yak calves. New born yak calves are protected against the threat of dogs, coyotes, wolves and other with the provision of shelter. For vaccination and other treatments a corral with a tunnel like passage is found in some places. For artificial insemination or mating to a particular bull a simple crush is often used to hold the female yak.

As discussed earlier, pens and enclosures are used only at night during the winter and spring. Location of the pens is usually at the campsite or close to the habitation of the herdsmen and their families. The pens are made up of various types of locally available materials and varying degree of permanence.

6.4.4.1 Turf pen

The semi-permanent pen is built to accommodate pack animals and bulls. The height of the turf walls is at least 60 cm, though usually higher. Open end of the pen faces towards sun and wall on the opposite site protect wind. As the structure is semi-permanent so needs repairing every year.

6.4.4.2 Wooden compound (or corral)

Wooden enclosure abundantly found where woods are easily available. Small wooden bars are used to make the compound where yak raiser hold hay. During the warm season, these wooden enclosures are used to keep the calves isolated from their dams at night, while the adults graze in preparation for milking the following morning. The wooden enclosures may be roofed or not. Wooden enclosures are often only used at the adjunct of mud pens and within its perimeter, where the availability of the wood is very scarce.

6.4.4.3 Mud pen

As the name indicates pens are constructed with a layer of clay on wooden boards knitted together with wicker. The dimension of the floor area is usually 15 x 15 m with a wall 1 - 1.2 m high. However, the size can be as large as 30 x 20 m. To protect the animals from the harsh wind an additional shelter area is constructed with one side facing to the sun. This type of pen is relatively permanent. When two or more mud pens built together, they are joined through a passage, having gates to restrain the animals within the particular pen. The passage is made up either by mud wall or wooden fence. If more number of pens are connected together, each pen is having the gate and the last pen will end in a long tunnel-like passage, which is either roofed or open. The tunnel is used to restrain the animals for vaccination, artificial insemination or treatment purpose.

6.4.4.4 Faeces pen

Fresh yak faeces are piled up in a layer of about 15 - 20 cm deep every day. The first layer freezes solid overnight before the second layer is added. Therefore, the pens can be completed within a few days. This type of pens are built temporarily and used only during the extreme cold season. As the temperature raises in the spring season the faeces starts thawing and pen become shattered. Similar type of pen again rebuilt in the next winter.

Faeces pens are of two types;

For adult animals : This type of pen comprises four walls to prevent wind and snow with a large area.

For calves : This type of pen is built like horseshoe-shaped foundation with a diameter of about 1 m, something like an upside-down earthen jar. The wall, opposite to the open end is made to protect the prevailing wind. A wooden stake is used to tether the calf. Hay is put inside the pen to make it warmer for the calf.

6.4.4.5 Other shelters

Small tents are made up on yak hair and the area varies from 10-20 m^2 which is surrounded by a stone wall of 1.5 m in height. Roof usually made up of boards or bark. They are found as a part of the permanent buildings of the campsites. This structure is also used for calf's shelter. They are also used by yak raisers and milkers and for processing milk and storing milk products.

6.4.5 Restraining

Some degree of control over the domestic animal's movement and activity is required for effectively manage the animal. Restraint practices when man first domesticated animals for food and fiber and as beasts of burden. Handling yak is similar to handling cattle and no special equipment is needed. Unlike other domesticated animals, yak only restraint at the time of milking or illness. The nostril is perforated to admit a rope tied with a slip-knot; by this means they are easily led. A local method, tying the fore limbs is most popular of restraining yak. Under this method of restraint, yak does not kick, although they make jumping movements. During the breeding season the breeding bulls become ferocious and it was quite difficult to separate the inseminated female yak from the bulls. Although, majority of the herders are of the view that the Chaleb (locally made raincoat to prevent natural service by breeding bulls) was very effective in preventing mating by breeding bulls, there were few herders questioning the efficacy of this method as some breeding bulls were able to remove it by use of their horns. Although yaks are maintained in free range system, they can be easily moved from one pasture to another, using a stick to guide them along.

6.4.6 Culling of yak

Culling is an important criterion to remove unproductive animals and to maintain the herd strength at desire level. Yak raises cull their animals when females are unproductive, breeding bulls are not at al used for breeding purpose, young male calves not necessary for breeding purpose. Some animals do not gain proper body before winter season due to many reason and they become weak. Yak raiser usually slaughter weak animals, just before winter, otherwise they will die during winter and coming spring. A yak cow is culled which provides 5-7 calves in her lifespan. Dressing percentage is 44-48%. Culling yak females with poor reproductive performance is not uncommon. Yak veal is very popular in some region and for that slaughtering the male calves at age of 6 months and poorly-developed female calves also reported.

6.4.7 Feeding Salt

Continuous leaching creates severe deficiency of minerals. Therefore, salt supplementation is a useful technique for better management of yaks. Yak does not take salt voluntarily and it has to be fed forcefully. The head is secured to the post by a short rope. The front and hind legs are tied together and the yaks brought to the ground on their sides. While one person holds the head and turns the mouth upwards, another person pours the salt down the animal's throat and follows it up with a mouthful of water to wash it down. Salt is fed thus to every animal monthly at the rate of 300-350 g per adult and 150- 200 g for yearlings.

6.4.8 Barter system of marketing of product of yak

Barter System is that system in which goods are exchanged for goods. Yak milk and milk product are not buying or selling through cash. Barter system is widely practiced. The barter system is prevalent between the yak herders and the food grain cultivators.

6.4.9 Yak management activity schedule

The various mangemental activities spread over different season. The activities start with the birth of the calves and ends with the production, processing and selling of products to the market. Unlike other domesticated species, their production is not so intensive. Mangemental activities are classified season-wise as discussed below:

- *Early summer*: As yak are seasonally poly-estrus, most the calving takes place in the summer months. Calving process is not problematic and finished within very short time. However, supervision and protection of the calves form the predators are necessary during and after parturition. This is main grazing season of the yak; therefore, they are adjusted and subdivided into different herd according to their age and productivity level, and allotted to the respective pasture. Those animals require castration; this is the ideal time for castration.

- *Middle of summer*: Yak does not tolerate heat. Therefore, they shed off their hair during summer months. This is the time when combing out down fibres and shearing is practiced. Parasitic load increases during this season. All the animals are dipped during this season as protection against external parasites. Vaccination against some diseases also done during this season. Milking operation is started one month after calving.
- *Late summer and autumn*: This is the mating season of yak. Females are mated to selected breeding male. Milking of the animals and processing of the milk continues during this season. As the winter season approaches, yak raiser harvest and store grasses for winter supplementation, especially for the sick and weak animals as well as for the pregnant animals.
- *Early winter*: Animals are returned from the very high altitude to the village site. Yak raisers engage in repairing of the pens and enclosures, where yak can be sheltered during winter. Yak raiser counts their animals. Unwanted and surplus stocks are culled. Usually animals are slaughtered for meat purpose.
- *Middle of winter*: Winter shelters are provided to the yak. Milking operation is stopped completely. Young calves are only allowed to suck as milk production decreases. Hardly 100 ml milk is available for the calf. If available supplements can be given to the pregnant yak to give priority to the developing foetus in the use of nutrients and body reserves.
- *Spring*: After a harsh long winter season imposes threat to the yak's life as feed resources are hardly available during this season. Females are very much susceptible to death as they either carry foetus or they are in lactating condition. Providing small amounts of supplementary grass as available (hay or possibly silage) and taking other measures to prevent death, particularly among the females. As the spring season ends the animals return to the pasture for grazing. Advanced pregnant animals are ready to give birth.

Table 6.3 : Month-wise different activities of yak husbandry

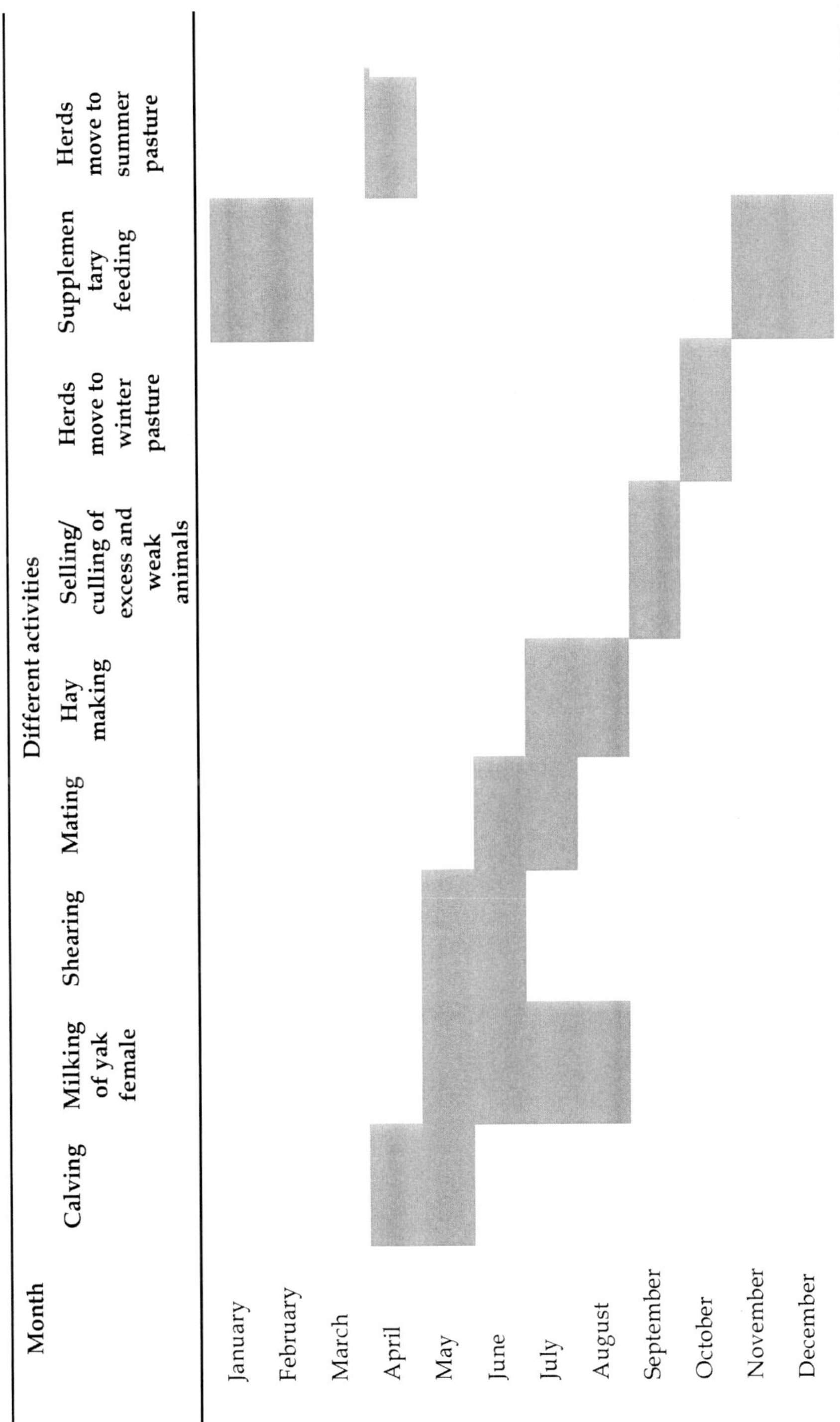

6.5 Dentition and determination of age

Like other domesticated mammals, yak has two types of dentition. Deciduous (D) or temporary or milk teeth appears in early life. It is gradually replaced by permanent dentition as yak grows. The deciduous dentition provides the young calves with a fully functional, though smaller set of teeth that can be accommodated by its small jaws. As the jaws grow longer, new permanent (P) teeth are added and the deciduous teeth are gradually replaced by permanent teeth. The deciduous or milk teeth are readily distinguished from the permanent teeth. The deciduous teeth are flat, long and wide at the initial stages but as age advances these become smaller and smaller in size until they are completely replaced by permanent teeth. The incisors are absent from the upper jaws of yak, their place being taken up by the "dental pad". They do not have any canine teeth. Incisors (I), and Premolars (P), with the exception of the first premolars are replaced. The molars (M), which erupt caudal to the premolars, are not present in the deciduous dentition. Replacement is gradual and follows a definite sequence, so that some deciduous and some permanent teeth are in use at the same time. As the developing permanent tooth pushes to the surface, it presses on the roots of the worn-out deciduous tooth and gradually cuts off its nutrition. The deciduous tooth becomes loose, eventually dies and is displaced.

The type of teeth is indicated by the first letter, and the number of teeth on one side of the upper jaw is indicated over the number of the same type of teeth on the lower jaw. Because the formula is for one side of the mouth the total number of teeth is the total in the formula x 2.

Deciduous (temporary) or milk teeth:

$$2\left(DI\frac{0}{4}DC\frac{0}{0}DP\frac{3}{3}\right) = \text{Total teeth -20}$$

Permanent teeth: $$2\left(I\frac{0}{4}C\frac{0}{0}P\frac{3}{3}M\frac{3}{3}\right) = \text{Total teeth -32}$$

Unlike cattle, new born yak calves do not have any incisors in the lower jaw. It appears gradually.

First week after birth : Incisor teeth are not present in the new born calf. The lower jaw at birth is a continuous red hard mass. In some cases, very small-pointed edges of dentine appear on the outer corner of both the first pair of incisors. Noticeable changes take place within seven days of birth. The first pair of incisors appears, the red hard mass starts showing demarcations and there are distinct signs for the appearance of incisor teeth.

Second week after birth : First pair of incisors completely exposed just after 7 days. One peculiar incidence occurs at this time. Third pair of incisors shows up a small pointed dentine spot in the red hard mass, although second and fourth pair of incisors is still embedded in the red hard mass.

Third week after birth : First pair of incisors continues to be broader and bigger, and becomes rounder as age progresses. At this age the second incisor has appeared but smaller than the third pair of incisors. Fourth pair of incisors is still embedded in the red hard mass. The red mass in between the incisor is retracted producing gaps between the incisors. At the completion of the third week there is a sign of eruption of the fourth pair of incisors.

Fourth week after birth : Fourth pair of incisors has just erupted and starts to grow. Rest of the incisors continues to be growing. The wide gaps between the incisors have been reduced to a great extent.

At the initial stage the upper edge of the incisors is sharp and uneven. As the age advances the uneven edges tend to become even. Replacement of deciduous teeth with the permanent teeth is just like cattle. By two years of age, all the milk teeth come out, the length and width varying from 1.2 to 1.6 cm and 0.6 to 1.1 cm, respectively.

Replacement of temporary teeth by permanent teeth : Around two years of age, the first pair of the temporary incisors is replaced by a pair of permanent incisors teeth. Similarly, the second pair of the incisors is replaced at three years of age. The third pair at fourth year and the fourth pair at fifth year of age are replaced. From five years onwards, the age is estimated by observing the wear and tear of the incisors, which are proportional to the age of the animal. A full-grown incisor is 2.0 cm in length and 1.4 cm in width, chiselled at the upper edge but angular inward. The chiselled edge becomes flattened and angular, wearing out as age advances (Pal *et al.*, 2000).

References

Bonnemaire J. 1984. Yak. In: Mason I.L. (ed), Evolution of domesticated animals. Longman, London, UK. pp. 39–45.

Cai Li. (1989). Sichuan yak. Chengdu, China, Sichuan Nationality Press.

Cai, L. and Wiener, G. (1995). The yak. Published by the Regional Office for Asia and the Pacific of the Food and Agriculture Organisation of the United Nations, Bangkok, Thailand pp. 1-105.

Dong Shikui et al. (2002). Availability and utilisation of shrubs as protein sources for yak grazing on alpine meadow on the Qinghai-Tibetan Plateau, China. Proceedings of the third international congress on yak, in Lhasa, China, 4-9 September 2000. International Livestock Research Institute (ILRI), Nairobi. pp. 273-279.

Dong, S.K., Long, R.J. and Dikken, G.D. (1999). Yak farming on the Qinghai-Tibetan Plateau of China. NCTR Livestock Newsletter . 1 and 2: 10- 14.

Indra, R. and Magash, A. (2000). Composition, quality and consumption of yak milk in Mongolia. Yak production in central Asian highlands Proceedings of the third international congress on yak held in Lhasa, P.R. China, 4–9 September.

Lensch, J. (1996). Krankheiten: In Der Yak (Bos grunniens) in Zentralasien (eds. Jurgen Lensch, Peter Schley and Rong-Chang Zhang). Duncker & Humblot. Berlin 1996, pp 237-246.

Liu Haibo. (1989). China Yakology. Sichuan Science and Technology Publishing House, Chengdu, China. pp. 119-123.

Miller, D.J. (1997). Conserving biological diversity in the HKH-Tibetan Plateau rangelands. Rangelands and pastoral development in the Hindu-Kush Himalayas - Proceedings of a regional experts Meeting (eds. D. J. Miller & S. R. Craig). ICIMOD, Kathmandu, Nepal.

Miller, D.J. (1996). Conserving and Managing Yak Genetic Diversity: An Introduction. In: Miller DJ, Craig SR, Rana GM (eds). Conservation and Management of Yak Genetic Diversity – Proc Workshop in ICIMOD, Oct.29-31, 1996, Kathmadu, Nepal.

Pal, R.N., Patnaik, S. and Mohanty, T.K. (2000). Dentition in yak. Yak production in central Asian highlands Proceedings of the third international congress on yak held in Lhasa, P.R. China, 4–9 September.

Sarbagishev, B.S., Rabochev, V.K. & Terebaev, A.I. (1989). Yaks. In Dmitriev N.G. & Emst, L.K. (ed), Animal genetic resources of the USSR. FAO Animal Production and Health Paper, No. 65, Rome. pp. 357-364.

Xu Guilin et al. (1983). Analysis of factors concerned with the milking performance and milk quality of yak. Journal of China Yak, 1: 21-29.

Yuan Youqing *et al.* (1994). Feed additive experiment to improve milk yield of yak. *Journal of China Yak*, 2: 11-13.

Zhang RC (1989). Yak of China. Lanzhou: Gansu Sci. Technol. Pub.House. pp. 1-98.

Zhang Rongchang (1989). China: the yak. Lanzhou, China, Gansu Scientific and Technology Press. pp 386.

Zhang Rongchang (1989). *China: the yak*. Lanzhou, China, Gansu Scientific and Technology Press. 386 pp.

Zhang Rongchang et al. (1986). Determination on the main composition in milk of Tianzhu White yak. Journal of China Yak, 2: 23-26.

Zhen Z. C. (1994). Population structure of yak herd in Naqu prefecture of Tibetan autonomy. Proceedings of the first international congress on yak. Journal of Gansu Agricultural University (Special issue June 1994), pp. 172-175.

Zhou, S.R. (1984). Study on the forage and feeding habits of yak. A research on the utilization and exploitation of grassland in the northwestern part of Sichuan Province. Chengdu: Sichuan National Publishing House. pp. 134-137.

Chapter 7

Production Performance

7.1 Growth

Growth may be defined as the increase in body mass and weight as a result of increase in structural tissues like muscle, bone and other organ and an important factor for determining the performance of a particular animal. Growth of an animal including human being are like a S shaped curve and called as sigmoid curve. From fetal to adult stage and thereafter is very much different, sometime slow, sometime fast and depends on so many factors like seasons which, along with the location, largely determine pasture growth and hence the feed supply to the dam as well as offspring. Age, sex, type or breeds of yak and herd management are among the other main causes of variation. The growth of the body weight as a whole is most commonly measured as an increase in weight. Size measures, such as height, chest girth and other body dimensions are also frequently employed. A combination of both weight size measures is much more useful than other alone. An animal may increase in weight through the deposition of fat without any increase in the structural tissues and organs which characterize growth. An animal which receiving feed with poor protein and energy may still exhibit increase in size due to skeletal growth. This is important for newborn yak, if calf born early in winter months, then insufficient milk and feed may lead to death of the calves.

In general, birth weight of yak calf is low, ranging from 9kg to 20kg and representing about 3 to 6 percent of adult weight. The relatively low birth weight is a consequence of a relatively short gestation length and the fact that in mid- and late pregnancy the yak, typically, has to exist on ground that is frozen and covered with ice and snow. In case of female, the birth weight is lower as compared to male and farmers select and fed the animals as per their body weight. Bat-Erdene (1988) reported the body measurements in Mongolian yak presented in table 7.1.

Table 7.1 : Body measurements of Yak.

Type of Animal	Height (cm)	Length (cm)	Heart girth (cm)
Bulls (n=5)	128.2 ± 0.96 (123 - 130)	152.4 ± 0.64 (146 - 162)	204.0 ± 0.83 (198 - 210)
Cows (n=160)	108.1 ± 0.41 (102 - 118)	120.9 ± 0.48 (114 - 132)	168.8 ± 0.79 (157 - 187)
Castrates (n=37)	127.4 ± 096 (115 - 139)	137.3 ± 0.12 (120 - 150)	189.1 ± 0.53 (177 - 219)

Although breed differences in birth weight may exist, it is not possible, as already mentioned, to differentiate between the effects of breed and those of location. Female calves are, on average, about 1 kg lighter at birth than the males. Zhang Rongchang (1989) observed that the height at wither may vary from 103 cm to around 138 cm, body length similarly, may vary from 113 cm to 173 cm, chest girth from 145 cm to 219 cm, body weight may vary from 193 kg to 600 kg depending on the species and location of the location of the yak. Linear body dimensions of yak at different ages as studied by (Zhong Guanghui *et al.,* 1996) and concluded that females at one year had reached between 5 percent and 10 percent more of their size at four years old than did the males. The results in the table 7.2 also show, as is well established in the literature, that some body parts such as height at withers and cannon-bone circumference, mature relatively earlier in life than do others such as chest depth and hip width.

Table 7.2 : Detail body measurements of yak of different ages.

Sex	Age (yr)	No.	Height at withers	Chest depth	Chest width	Hip width	Heart girth	Cannon bone circumf.	Rump length	Body length
M	1	226	94.8 ± 20.7	44.4 ± 6.0	20.1 ± 2.7	23.8 ± 3.0	119.7 ± 12.9	13.7 ± 1.0	31.9 ± 3.5	99.8 ± 8.3
	2	155	104.4 ± 5.5	53.9 ± 5.4	23.9 ± 3.9	27.8 ± 3.3	138.5 ± 10.2	15.4 ± 1.1	36.1 ± 2.6	114.8 ± 7.9
	3	116	110.9 ± 5.7	58.6 ± 5.1	25.8 ± 3.5	30.4 ± 3.3	153.6 ± 13.0	16.5 ± 1.1	38.9 ± 3.8	124.5 ± 12.9
	4	91	122.4 ± 8.6	67.9 ± 7.8	32.3 ± 8.2	36.9 ± 6.8	177.6 ± 18.6	18.8 ± 1.9	45.0 ± 5.3	140.2 ± 12.6
F	1	220	91.5 ± 6.3	43.8 ± 5.3	20.2 ± 5.7	23.2 ± 3.0	117.4 ± 11.0	13.4 ± 1.0	30.4 ± 3.5	97.4 ± 8.7
	2	157	101.6 ± 5.3	51.6 ± 4.3	23.7 ± 4.4	27.6 ± 2.8	134.3 ± 13.7	14.7 ± 1.0	34.9 ± 3.9	111.4 ± 11.4
	3	181	107.1 ± 4.9	56.2 ± 3.7	24.5 ± 3.2	30.7 ± 3.6	147.6 ± 9.7	15.7 ± 0.9	37.5 ± 2.4	120.0 ± 6.7
	4	190	110.8 ± 6.3	58.9 ± 6.0	25.4 ± 5.2	32.2 ± 3.4	153.4 ± 11.7	16.1 ± 0.7	39.0 ± 2.2	126.1 ± 7.6
	5	160	112.1 ± 4.5	60.9 ± 3.2	25.8 ± 3.9	33.4 ± 3.4	158.1 ± 9.7	16.3 ± 0.6	40.3 ± 2.2	127.5 ± 11.2

In yak, as in other bovines, the linear body dimensions show less seasonal variation in size than is found for body weight. Relatively early-maturing dimensions that are largely a function of skeletal size, such as height at withers, show less variability in size over the seasons than dimensions that mature later and also include, in the measurement, a greater proportion of muscle and fat (e.g. heart girth). Ma Zongxiang and Dou Yaozong (1981) studied the monthly change of live weight, monthly gain and daily gain of calves in cold and warm seasons in Tibet and observed (table 7.3) that growth during cold season goes negatively as compared to warm season. This of course an effect of availability of nutrient for growth was most important.

Table 7.3 : Growth rate of yak calf at different seasons.

Season	Month	Age of calf (months)	Live weight (kg)	Monthly gain (kg)	Daily gain (g)
Warm season	July	2	21.1 ± 1.5	-	-
	August	3	28.4 ± 2.0	6.3 ± 0.6	213.7 ± 21.1
	September	4	35.2 ± 2.6	5.1 ± 0.8	180.3 ± 19.4
Cold season	October	5	39.0 ± 3.1	5.2 ± 1.0	168.2 ± 11.7
	November	6	38.3 ± 1.8	-0.6 ± 0.3	-23.0 ± 5.1
	December	7	37.2 ± 2.7	-0.4 ± 0.3	-13.3 ± 3.0
	January	8	37.0 ± 4.0	-0.8 ± 0.4	-31.1 ± 1.2
	February	9	37.5 ± 2.3	0.5 ± 0.3	16.2 ± 2.4
	March	10	36.1 ± 1.4	-0.7 ± 0.4	-23.0 ± 3.0
	April	11	37.4 ± 1.3	0.5 ± 0.2	17.0 ± 4.0
Warm season	May	12	32.3 ± 2.4	-5.4 ± 0.2	-188.7 ± 24.1
	June	13	38.5 ± 3.0	8.0 ± 1.2	250.1 ± 25.0
	July	14	45.3 ± 3.4	5.3 ± 1.0	184.5 ± 14.2

Pourochottamane *et al.* (2007) observed the growth pattern of yak supplementing concentrate mixture upto 4 years of age and concluded that the body weight of male and female calves were almost similar until six months of age, only from the 15th month onwards was the difference in body weight between male and female calves evident, however, the difference was not statistically significant up to 18 months of age. The body weight at 24, 30, 36, 42 and 48 months of age were around 223, 266, 281, 313 and 357 kg, respectively in males and 190, 217, 237.33, 245 and 258 kg, respectively in female yak and the differences were statistically significant ($P<0.05$). The authors also concluded that three-fourth of the adult body weight was attained by the female yaks by two years of age, whereas males attained this by 30 months of age. Unlike in traditional yak rearing system where adult body weight is reached by 5 to 6 years of age, under the semi-range system of management, the adult body weight is reached by around 4 years of age.

7.1.1 Factors affecting growth

Supplementary feeding of the dams were small but positive both on birth weight and daily weight gain and may have reached statistical significance, according to the report of Wen Yongli *et al.* (1993). Farmers provide also winter supplementation for better milk production and dam survivability. National Research Centre on Yak, Dirang, Arunachal Pradesh, India has come to the conclusion that nutritional intervention in terms of mineral supplementation resulted in decreased age at puberty (from 3.5 to 4.5 years to 1.5 to 2.5 years), increased adult body weight (female: from 150-200 kg to 250-350 kg and male: from 250-300 to 450-550 kg), and better reproductive efficiency. Effect of urea supplementation at different levels, over a basal diet of finger millet straw, in yaks on DM intake and nutrient utilization was studied by the Centre, and reported that there was no significant effect on DM intake and DM digestibility co-efficients. However, TDN and DCP contents significantly increased with the increase in level of urea supplementation. The preliminary findings showed that concentrate supplementation in feed have a significant effect on average daily weight gain than that of control group in yaks. Ghosh and Bandopadhayay (2007) reported that traditional yak farming suffers a set back due to inadequate feeding resulted in herbage and nutritional deficiencies, this resulted in poor body weight gain, infertility or low production. Ghosh and Bandopadhyay (2008) reported that supplementary feeding with concentrate scientifically, improved daily gain in the yak of Arunachal Pradesh. Pourochottamane *et al.* (2007) observed the growth pattern of yak supplementing concentrate mixture at 50 and 30 percent of DM intake, daily body weight gain ($P<0.01$) and feed conversion efficiency ($P<0.05$) were significantly higher in animals fed with the high concentrate diet. An insignificant difference in the dry matter intake was observed between the 2 groups. They concluded that the higher rate of concentrate supplementation was beneficial in improving the growth performance of male yak calves.

Parity and age of cow : Both parity and age of yak dam have effects on the birth weight of their calves, as shown in the following table and as widely reported in studies on ordinary cattle elsewhere. Chen Zhihua *et al.* (1994) reported that dams with 4th and 5th parity are good for birth weight of the calves and calves born in early parities are lighter in weight. Farmers observation is that 1st calves from are weaker and very much prone to disease and in most of the cases dies.

Table 7.4 : Effects of parity and of age of yak cow on the birth weight of her calf.

Parity of dam	No. of cows	Deviation of birth weight (kg)	Age of dam (years)	No. of cows	Deviation of birth weight (kg)
1	37	-0.02	4	33	-0.52
2	27	-0.34	5	9	-0.24
3	26	-0.26	6	3	-0.23
4	28	-0.90	7	20	0.62
5	20	0.81	8	21	0.25
6	18	0.71	9	32	0.54
			10	38	-0.42

Body weight and body condition of the dam : Not surprisingly, farmers aware about the body condition and weight of the dam during and just after birth affects the birth weight of the calves. They fed their animals depends on their body weight during the winter months for better productivity of milk and dam performance. There are several other factors like month of calving i.e., winter calves survives less as compared to summer one. Chen Zhihua *et al.* (1994) observed that date and month of birth of the calves have an impact on birth weight (highly significant, $P<0.01$). Typically, weight gain in a healthy calf reared by its dam is almost linear over the first six months of life, but declines with the approach of winter; this is followed by some loss in weight over the first winter and spring. Thereafter, in the second warm season, there is again a rapid gain in weight followed, once more, by a loss in weight over the next cold season. Management system followed at the farmers may also affect the growth of the calves which may be attributed by availability of milk to the calf, nutrient supply to the dam for milk precursor synthesis and weaning of the calf from the dam. Traditionally the calves are not separated from the dam until it becomes mature. Zhang Rongchang (1989) observed that the dam milked once a day or not milked had grown better that dam milked twice, indicted the importance of milk the yak calf. Las factor which is the breed and location, sex also have the effect on growth of the calf, i.e., male calves have better chance to grow faster than its female counterpart and alpine yak (viz., Juilong) grow more faster than other breeds. The same is true for location of the yak as changing the place from one to another the breed may not exhibit its optimum production potential perhaps due to adaptation characteristics.

7.2 Meat Production

Meat production is the result of growth of the animal and it is assumed that any animal attaining growth early are good for the purpose. As meat production is the result of growth of the animals, farmer fed their animal so that dressing percentage and meat yield go higher. Meat from yak is derived from surplus males, often the castrated steers, and also from females, usually at the end of their useful reproductive life, or at the end of their time as milk-producers. In India, mostly slaughtered on some socio-religious occasions and especially in the winter months when vegetables, milk and meat are scarce in the region.

7.2.1 Meat quantity

The major factor contributing to meat output is the body weight of the animal at the time of slaughter. Thus, the factors associated with variation in growth, discussed earlier, all influence the amount of meat produced. Grass growth, as affected by season and location, is the major contributor, along with breed, age and sex of the animal. Seasonal changes in body weight, shown earlier in this chapter, clearly affect meat output. In practice, animals intended for meat are slaughtered, whenever possible, mostly in the winter when other food items are rarely available. There are several factors which affect the meat production in yak discussed below.

*Breed and location:*There is much variation in the slaughter quality of different breeds of yak at different locations in terms of dressing percentage, ratios of lean to bone and loin-eye area etc. Depending on the breed and location of yak, dressing percent may vary from 32 to 60, whereas, loin eye area may vary from around 30 to 86 sq cm. Live weight at slaughter may also vary depending on breed, location and management practice at farm level. Smirnov *et al.* (1990), the low dressing percentage was attributed to the slaughter of young male yak at what was considered the wrong age - two years old. There was also substantial variation in loin eye area. It should be noted, however, that in some instances the numbers on which the means are based are very small. Most of the information should be regarded as indicative of the range of values found in yak rather than definitive of the merits of any particular class or location of yak.

7.2.2. Effect of age and sex

It is observed that the for steer yak to have the higher live weights and carcass weights at slaughter relative to females and perhaps higher dressing percentages. However, there is not a consistent finding. Also, a report by Ji Qiumei *et al.* (2000b) indicated that in one of two groups (Jiali yak), dressing percentages and lean/bone ratio were similar in the two sexes and in the other group (Sibu yak) the females were the better in these traits from the data on a herd of 3142 farmed yaks in the northern Caucasus. They also concluded that meat produced by the yaks had better flavour and tenderness than that from local cattle. It was also suggested that the optimum age at slaughter for (male) yaks is 2.5-3 yr. Jialin *et al.* (1998b) reported that dressing percent was similar at 6 months (between male and female) and 18 months age (between male and female) wild yak and crossbred yak whereas live weight, carcass weight and meat weight was significantly higher in 18 months age group. Meat to bone ratio, loin eye area chunk and dorsal meat, rib weight, shank weight, loin weight and rump weight were also higher in 18 months age group. Brisket weight was though similar statistically. Chinese workers reported that in a trial in Sichuan province, entire male yak from the age of 1.5 - 4.5 years and thereafter, yak steers to the age of 20.5 years were chosen at random from yak herds in the same area and kept under year-round grazing without supplementary feeding. All the animals were slaughtered at the Animal Husbandry and Veterinary Station in Kangdin county of Sichuan at the end of autumn, in their fattest condition. In spite of the small number of animals involved, the trends shown in following table 7.5 indicated that the dressing percentage increased with age (and live weight) up to six and a half years and declined somewhat thereafter. However, the castration of males after the age of four and a half years and the subsequent switch to steers could be an important factor in the larger increase in dressing percentage noted between the ages of four and a half and five and a half years. Variation among the steers above the age of 16.5 years showed no clear trends (the data for these ages have been pooled).

Table 7.5 : Dressing percentage of yak males and steers, according to age at slaughter

Age (years)	Sex	No.	Live weight (kg)	Dressing (percent)
1.5	Male	2	55	37.6
2.5	Male	2	105	44.0
3.5	Male	2	182	47.6
4.5	Male	2	234	49.6
5.5	Steer	2	370	55.8
6.5	Steer	3	401	56.2
7.5	Steer	4	407	53.9
10.5	Steer	1	409	51.7
11.5	Steer	2	417	55.0
14.5	Steer	3	406	52.3
16.5-20.5	Steer	10	413	53.4

7.2.3 Meat quality

Yak meat is fine textured and scarlet in colour. It is regarded as very palatable, but muscular marbling is poor. It is rich in myoglobins and has a flavour similar to game. Among local people yak meat has been prized above that of ordinary cattle since ancient times. Several workers reported the yak meat composition is summarized in table 7.6 yak meat from different breed and location. Smirnov *et al.* (1990) observed the slaughter quality of yak cow and bull and reported that average pre-slaughter weight was 287 and 205 kg for cows and bulls, respectively. Carcass yield was 45.4 and 39.5 percent, yield of perivisceral fat was 3.2 and 0.8 percent and carcasses contained 83.4 and 79.7 percent lean and 16.6 and 20.3 percent bone, respectively. Longissimus dorsi contained water 75.2 and 76.3, protein 21.8 and 22.0, fat 2.0 and 0.6 and ash 1.10 and 1.11 percent; tryptophan 435 and 407 and hydroxyproline 62.3 and 74.1 mg/100 g. They also opined that yak meat had excellent cooking qualities.

Besides location, sex, age and breed, the rearing or management especially the nutrient intervention of the animals, which is reflected in body condition, must be expected to affect the meat composition of yak. Zhang Rongchang (1989) indicates the relationship between rearing treatment and meat composition of yak (table 7.7). It can be seen that dry matter, fat and energy in yak steer meat increased with the improved feeding level.

Table 7.6 : Composition of yak steer meat (percent)

Province/ country	Breed or Location	No.	Age (years)	Meat from	Dry matter	Protein	Fat	Ash	Ca	P	Source
Sichuan	Maiwa	7	1.5	Rib 9-11	25.8	21.5	3.3	1.04			Cai Li *et al.*, 1984
Xingjiang	Bazhou	2	2.5	Rib 9-11	24.7	21.2	2.0	1.07			Wei Ronglu *et al.*, 1981
Gansu	Tianzhu White	3	4.5	Rib 9-10	33.8	20.0	11.9	0.87	0.02	0.14	Pu Ruitang *et al.*, 1987
				Loin eye	23.7	21.3	1.4	1.05	0.02	0.20	Pu Ruitang *et al.*,1987
Qinghai	Qinghai	NA	4.5	Back, rib	25.9	22.1	2.1	1.61	0.03	0.20	Lei Huanzhang *et al.*, 1983
		NA	Over 6	Back, rib	26.8	22.3	2.8	1.68	0.02	0.24	Lei Huanzhang *et al.*, 1983
	Domestic yak	6	0.5	Rib 9-11	25.8	22.6	3.3	1.04	-	-	Jialin *et al.*, 1998b
		3	1.5	Rib 9-11	31.1	22.6	7.9	1.17	-	-	Jialin *et al.*, 1998b
	Wild yak x domestic yak crosses	6	0.5	Rib 9-11	27.5	22.7	3.6	1.05	-	-	Jialin *et al.*, 1998b
		3	1.5	Rib 9-11	31.1	22.2	5.9	1.09	-	-	Jialin *et al.*, 1998b
Tibet	Pali	6	Adult	Rib 9-11	44.1	17.8	25.3	0.84	0.020	-	Ji Qiumei *et al.*, 2000c
				Loin eye	25.8	22.6	2.1	1.03	0.032	-	Ji Qiumei *et al.*, 2000c
Mongolia	Mongolia	?	Adult	Rib 9-11	27.2	18.8	5.0	0.92	-	-	Zhang Rongchang, 1989

Table 7.7 : Composition of yak steer meat (percent) under different rearing treatments in Kyrgyzstan

Group	Age (month)	No.	Live weight (kg)	Dressing (percent)	Dry matter (percent)	Protein (percent)	Fat (percent)	Ash (percent)	Energy (MJ/kg)
I	19	22	234	44.0	26.8	23.0	2.4	1.1	4.9
II	19	22	258	46.3	27.4	22.8	3.6	1.1	5.3
III	19	22	275	49.8	28.9	22.2	5.7	1.0	6.0

I: suckling the (milked) dam; II: milk with artificial rearing, III: milk with artificial rearing together with supplementation in the cold season

Zi *et al.* (2004) observed the estimated live weights, carcass characteristics, the proximate composition and amino-acid composition of the whole rib cut of the $10^{th}/12^{th}$ thoracic vertebrae have been determined for Jiulong-yak and reported that the animal grows rapidly up to puberty at 2-3 years of age. At those ages, females reached 143 kg and 184 kg respectively, which was 60 to 80 percent of their mature weight at 6 to 7 yr old, then the rate of growth significantly slowed down. Males continued to rapidly increase body weight until an older age possibly due to the selection procedures. Dressing percentage and rib eye area ranged from 48.53-55.04 percent and 48.02-68.56 sq cm respectively, both of which differed by age and sex. The $10^{th}/12^{th}$ rib-cut contained 24.99-31.93 percent dry matter; 19.98-22.58 percent protein; 2.52-10.86 percent fat and 0.93-1.00 percent ash. Meat from females and steers contained a higher percentage of fat than those from bulls. The pH of muscle *Longissimus dorsi* measured at 24 h post-mortem ranged from 5.84-6.11. Amino acid composition was similar to that for other red meat, except for a lower content of methionine (1.26 g/100 g meat). The results indicated that yak meat can make a valuable contribution to the diets for the highlanders. Luo *et al.* (2006) reported that the meat of the adult male yak was 7.35 mg/kg higher in calcium ($P < 0.05$) and 124 mg/kg higher in phosphorus ($P < 0.01$) than that of the adult female yak. There was an obvious difference in zinc content, and there was also a significant difference for copper and sulfur between adult male and female yaks ($P < 0.01$). Iron was 8.85 mg/kg higher in semi-wild yaks than in domestic yaks, but there were no differences for other minerals. Further, they showed that the data showed that introducing wild yak's blood did not result in a quality change in the domestic yak meat. Yak meat from Qinghai Plateau has the characteristics of being non-polluted and rich in amino acids in comparison with local yellow cattle meat. The ratio of essential to nonessential amino acids was found to be between 0.6:1 and 0.8:1.

7.3 Draught Performance

The yak is widely used for draught purposes at the high altitudes where it makes its home - and not only as the pack animal for much publicized, Himalayan mountaineering expeditions, known worldwide. The yak has strong limbs, small, solid hooves with hard edges and a narrow hoof fork. These attributes help the yak to walk in dangerous places and over marshland and to climb over steep mountains. It can open up a path with its head and its hooves for people to follow, and it can swim across rapids. In difficult terrain it is said to be safer to ride on a yak than on a horse, as the yak will not readily panic, for example in swampy ground. Since ancient times, the yak has been known in the mountainous regions of China and surroundings as the 'boat of the plateau'.

Most of the yak used for draught are steers. The draught animals are used mainly for riding and as pack animals. Though in recent times, yak crossbreds and yak steers are used for ploughing in regions where tractor can not reach. Farmers also sing a melodious song to encourage the animal. Yak races are one of the games at folk festivals much loved by Tibetan people. In semi-agricultural areas yak are also used for ploughing and other cultivation. Yak have great endurance; they will, for example, carry loads over long distances for two or three days without water or feed. In other circumstances, the yak may be required to carry loads during the day, with the opportunity to graze only at night, for as long as a month at a stretch. Joshi (1982) also refers to the use of yak and hybrids for threshing grain in parts of Tibet by driving muzzled animals backward and forward over sheaves spread out on a hard floor. Yak can be ridden by the herders on the high plateau. A study by Lei Huanzhang *et al.* (1985) showed three Plateau-type yak were ridden on fairly even grassland at an elevation of 4400 m for 500 m in 2.13 minutes. Their respiration, pulse and body temperature recovered in just over 25 minutes. National Research Centre on Yak, Dirang, Arunachal Pradesh, India examined to observe the effect of castration on pack performance (Kataktalware *et al.,* 2007). The experimental animals were comprised of 6 castrated and 6 non-castrated male yaks of similar ages. The exercise schedule comprised of walking uphill for 5 km with a load of 10 percent body weight of animals for 4 weeks. The results showed that immediately after exercise, the body temperature and respiration rate of castrated and non-castrated animals varied significantly (P<0.05). However, post-exercise observations on all clinical parameters did not depict significant differences. Similarly, it was observed that there were insignificant differences between the castrated and non-castrated animals in terms of any of the haematological parameters. It was concluded that there was no adverse effect of castration on the pack performance of yak.

7.3.1 Milk Production

Milk may be defined as the whole lacteal secretion obtained by complete milking of one or more healthy lactating females at least after 72 h of parturition. Milk from the dam is nature's gift to the offspring though W D Hoard rightly said that 'the cow is the foster mother of the human race'. From the day of the ancient Hindoo to this time have the thoughts of man turned to this kindly and beneficient creature as one of the chief sustaining forces of human life. Milk is a white opaque fluid with some exceptions where it is tinge yellowish particularly in some breeds. Because of content of almost all essential nutrients (except iron), milk is being used throughout the world for feeding infants and as supplement to the diets of children and adults. In milk fat along with some fat soluble vitamins are present as an emulsion (colloidal dispersion of one liquid in another immiscible or partially miscible liquid), protein along with some mineral matters in colloidal suspensions, lactose together with some water soluble minerals and vitamins are in true solutions. The main constituents of milk are depicted diagrammatically below.

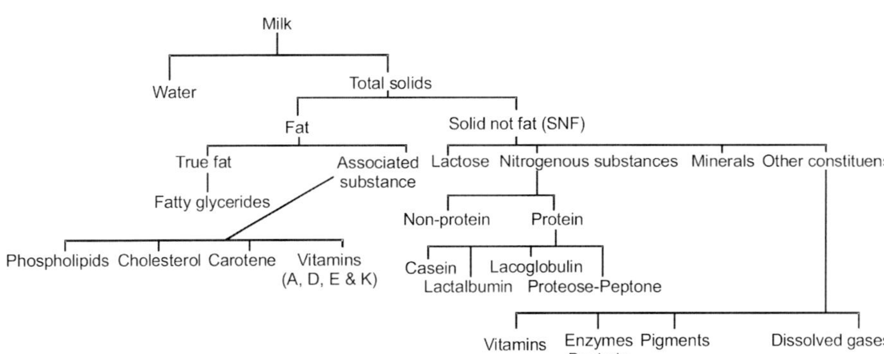

Though there, at present, no breed or strain of yak developed especially for milk production. All breeds are kept, to a greater or lesser extent, to produce milk, in addition to their other uses and products. Yak milk is creamy white in colour, having thick consistency and peculiar yak hair or sweat odour which is more prevalent in winter season. Preparation of byproducts like paneer, an acid coagulant milk product from yak milk is an excellent way to overcome the problem of inaesthetic perception. This is though, not a common practice among the farmers. Traditionally paneer is prepared with full fat resulting in rich flavour, soft consistency, lower sliceability and early spoilage. Yak milk paneer having very high fat needs very special attention due to growing concerns of health related problems even in the rural masses arising from consumption high milk fat contents. Poorest of poor farmer want to fetch more money from his products and this is only possible when low fat paneer is prepared. Kandeepan *et al.* (2010) reduced the level of fat to increase the SNF and then prepared paneer, resulted in lower paneer yield, reduced the microbial content of paneer while the paneer had low fat content with improved body and texture. Sarmah *et al.* (2009) reported that low fat (3 percent) milk from yak was having similar sensory scores and excellent organoleptic attributes with high fat milk (4 and 5 percent). So milk byproducts may also be prepared at farmers level for economic upliftment of the people.

Mammals have the mammary gland or udder from which milk is secreted. Mammary glands are the modified sweat gland and are located outside the abdominal cavity. Its only connection with the abdominal cavity is through inguinal canal a potential tube about 4 inches long in cow, through which blood and lymph vessels and nerve fibres leave the abdominal cavity to enter the udder. The right and left halves indicated by the inter-mammary groove. The fore and rear quarters may be smoothly joined or may be demarketed by varying degrees of grooving. Yak udders are small as compared to dairy cattle, not well developed. Measurements in Sichuan showed an udder circumference in multiparous females of 55 cm and an udder depth of between 2 and 3 cm in 60 females measured in Qinghai (Zang Yinsong, 1985). Usually the two rear quarters hold more milk than the two forequarters. The forequarters are generally supposed to hold about 45 percent of the milk and the sphincter muscles of the yak teats are strong and hard squeezing is needed to extract milk. The teats are normally squeezed between the fingers.

Colostrum, on the other hand, is the first secretion from the mother after giving birth of its child and richer in most nutrients apart from lactose and fat. Since placental barrier does not allow to pass antibodies and neonate depends on colostrum for passive immunity solely. Colostrum of ruminants contains trypsin inhibitor which protects the immunoglobulins from digestion. Within three to four days after parturition milk losses its colostral properties and becomes normal. Total solids in colostrum is much higher than milk especially due to protein and ash content. A comparison of composition between colostrum and normal milk of yak as studied by Liu Haibo (1989) and Zhang Rongchang (1989) is shown in table 7.8 and clearly indicated that the difference between colostrum and milk exists as in other species of animals.

Table 7.8 : Composition of Yak Milk vs. Colostrum

Species	No.	Milk type	Milk solid (percent)	Fat (percent)	Protein (percent)	Lactose (percent)	Ash (percent)
Yak	17	Colostrum	32.0 - 34.5	13.2 -15.8	15.1 -17.1	1.7 - 1.9	0.9 - 1.1
Yak	33	Normal milk	16.9 - 17.7	5.5 - 7.2	4.9 - 5.3	4.5 - 5.0	0.8 - 0.9

7.3.2 Milk from different species

Milk from different species are different based on their neonates need and for survival in a particular environment. For example, fat content of grey seal is more than 52 percent, where as in sheep, goat and cattle its only 3-5 percent while buffalo and yak have 7-10 percent required for nourishing and optimum growth of their offspring. The following table 7.9 shows the composition of milk from different species.

Table 7.9 : Milk composition (percent) of different species

Species	Fat	Protein	Lactose	Ash	Total solids
Indian buffalo	7.4	3.8	4.9	0.78	16.8
Camel	4.9	3.7	5.1	0.70	14.4
Cow					
Sahiwal	4.5	3.3	5.0	0.66	13.3
Gir	4.7	3.3	4.9	0.66	13.3
Red Sindhi	4.9	3.4	4.9	0.70	13.7
Holstein	3.5	3.1	4.9	0.70	12.2
Jersey	5.5	3.9	4.9	0.70	15.0
Goat	3.5	3.1	4.6	0.79	12.0
Sheep	5.3	5.5	4.6	0.90	16.3
Rat	14.8	11.3	2.9	1.50	31.7
Elephant	15.1	4.9	3.4	0.76	26.9
Whale	34.8	13.6	1.8	1.60	51.2
Grey Seal	53.2	11.2	2.6	0.70	67.7
Yak	10.9	4.0	3.5	0.98	19.3
Human	4.5	1.1	6.8	0.20	12.6

Source: Textbook of Animal Husbandry, G C Banerjee (8th Ed).Oxford & IBH Publishing Co, New Delhi

Under Indian condition Mondal and Pal (1996) examined 36 samples of yak milk, which were all mastitis test-negative and varied in colour from yellowish white to golden yellow, had the following composition specific gravity- 1.030; titratable acidity-0.29 percent; pH- 6.0; total solids-15.63 percent; SNF-7.05 percent; fat-8.6; lactose-4.52 g/dl, ash-0.4 percent.

7.3.3 Milk biosynthesis

Most of the organic constituents of milk arise from specific synthetic processes of the mammary gland, representing products which are not found elsewhere in nature. As an aid to a consideration of physiology involved and the chemical changes which takes place, representative data are depicted in the following table 7.10 on the composition of milk and of the blood plasma of cow. Some constituents are directly coming to milk from blood and some are synthesized in the mammary gland tissue. Certain constituents including lactose, casein and some of the fatty acids are the synthetic products of the gland while others like minerals and vitamins are directly coming from blood. The milk of an individual animal is known to contain constant composition but there are periodic fluctuations especially fat which changes over the course of lactation. The factors affecting yield and composition is discussed later in this chapter.

Table 7.10 : Composition of blood plasma and milk of cow

Blood plasma		Milk	
Constituent	**Percent**	**Constituent**	**Percent**
Water	91.0	Water	87.0
Glucose	0.05	Lactose	4.90
		Casein	2.90
Serum albumin	3.20	Lactaclbumin	0.52
Serum globulin	4.40	Lactoglobulin	0.20
Neutral fat	0.06	Neutral fat	3.75
Phospholipids	0.24	Phospholipids	0.10
Calcium	0.009	Calcium	0.12
Phosphorus	0.011	Phosphorus	0.10
Sodium	0.34	Sodium	0.05
Potassium	0.03	Potassium	0.15
Chlorine	0.35	Chlorine	0.11
Citric acid	Trace	Citric acid	0.20

Source: Animal Nutrition, 7th Ed, Maynard *et al.*TMH edition.

7.3.4 Precursors of milk

There are differences in milk and blood component and as discussed some of the constituents synthesized in the mammary tissue.

Protein: It is made up of a number of specific proteins, with casein being the most important component. Casein, lactalbumin, lactoglobulin are not present in blood, these must be synthesized from blood precursors. These three components comprise about 90-95 percent of total nitrogen in milk. The immunoglobulins and serumalbumin appear to be identical in blood and milk are thus diffuses in milk in unchanged form from blood.

Lactose: Its accepted that glucose is the principal blood precursor of lactose. In the mammary gland it is synthesized and the steps are shown below

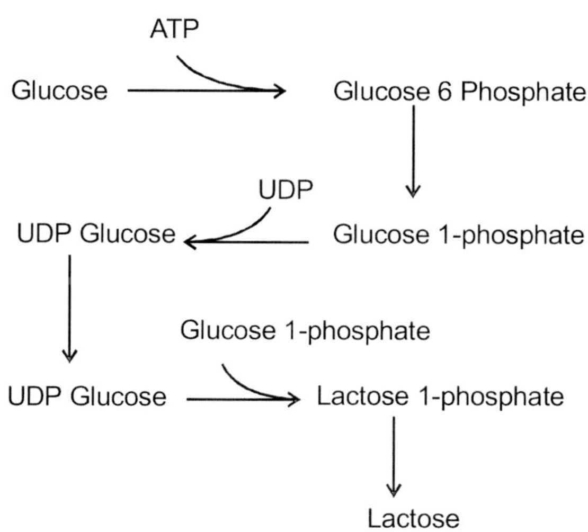

Lactose biosvnthesis

Fats/ Lipids: The fatty acids in milk occur almost entirely as triglycerides, in contrast to the situation in plasma where they present largely as phospholipids. Glucose is the carbon source for fatty acid synthesis in nonruminants while in ruminants i.e., cattle, sheep, goat, buffalo, yak, mithun etc. acetate and â-hydroxy- butyrate from rumen fermentation. This volatile fatty acids are originated from fibre fermentation in rumen and thus one can expect less milk fat from the animals fed rich in grain or concentrate feeds. Fatty acids having more than 16 carbon originates from blood, though polyunsaturated fatty acids are the fermentation end product directly coming to milk. Now a days, scientists are involves in production and somebody have partially succeed in production of functional food of milk rich in omega-3 fatty acid and other components which has a health benefit effect. Pathway of milk fat synthesis is shown below.

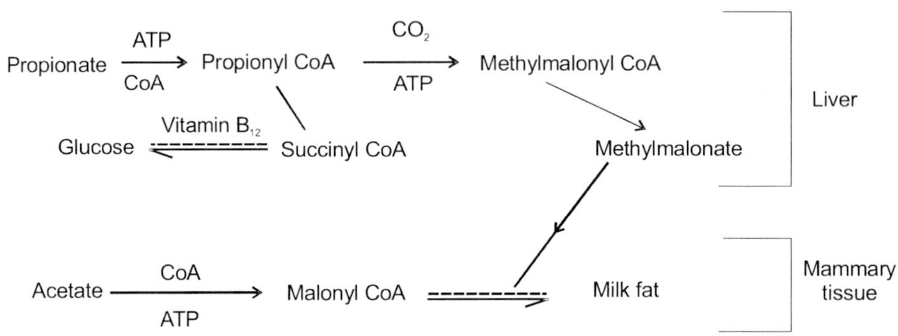

Minerals, pigments and vitamins: Over thirty minerals have been found in milk, many of them present in traces. Thus the list of double the number which have been found to be essential nutrients. They all are from blood plasma. Many of the minerals of milk such as calcium, potassium, sodium, chlorine, iron, nickel, magnesium, and phosphorus are affected very little by the dietary intake. Other minerals including zinc, cobalt, copper, manganese may be lowered by a deficient diet to the dam. Iodine content of milk highly variable depending on dietary intake of the mineral. Milk is well protected against cadmium, mercury and selenium. While there is a positive correlation between dietary intake and milk concentration, the transfer to milk is very inefficient. Milk contains both fat and water soluble vitamins and pigments like xanthophyll, carotene. Of the fat soluble vitamins precursor of vitamin A is the principal one in the cow milk. Chlorophyll is destroyed in digestive tract, some amount of xanthophyll may be seen in milk. The principal water soluble vitamin is riboflabin and all these are coming directly from blood.

7.4 Factors affecting milk composition

The variation in composition and daily yield of milk is a regular phenomenon in any milking animals. Broadly, the factors which are responsible for such variations can be either physiological (which will be governed by genetic make up) or environmental (age, parity, pregnancy, nutritional status, disease, management of animals/ farm, microclimate, weather conditions etc). Variation in the composition of milk may result from one or more causes which discussed below.

a. *Breed*: The composition of milk varies with a number of non-nutritional factors, one of the most marked being the effect of breed. The within breed variation in milk composition is also very common. The fat and crude protein content of milk are related inversely to the lactation yield. Lactose value tend to be slightly higher in milk from breed with high fat content and thus the SNF (protein + lactose + ash) content are also higher. Because of this fairly close relationship between fat and SNF content the selection dam for milk production, a higher fat content should also ensure a high SNF content. The table 7.11 shows the different breed producing milk and fat content.

Table 7.11 : Milk yield and fat percentage of yak females of different breeds at various locations of China

Yak breed or yak location*	Month of measurement	N.	Average daily yield (kg)	Estimated lactation yield, kg, (in days)	Fat (percent)	Source
Tianzhu White	5 - 10	223	2.3 ± 0.5	304 (135)	6.8	Zhang Rongchang, 1989
Huanhu	6 - 10	96	3.0 ± 0.3	487 (153)	6.4	Zhang Rongchang, 1989
Guoluo	7 - 11	20	1.0 ± 0.2	162 (153)	6.6	Li Quan *et al.*, 2000b
Maiwa	4, 7	20	1.8	365 (150)	6.8	Chen Xiafei *et al.*, 1981
Jiulong	7, 8	93	2.8 ± 0.2	414 (150)	5.7	Cai Li *et al.*, (1980a)
Pali	7 - 9	19	2.7 ± 0.3	280 (105)		Zhang Rongchang, 1989
Jiali		48	0.8 ± 0.2	148 (180)	6.8	Ji Qiumei *et al.*, 2000a
Sibu		36	0.9 ± 0.1	180 (180)	7.5	Ji Qiumei *et al.*, 2000a
Zhongdian	5, 7, 11	81	1.1 ± 0.2	192 (180-210)	6.2	Zhang Rongchang, 1989

b. *Changes in normal lactation*: Lactation period of animal is the period from the time animal gives birth to a young till she goes dry. It is very different in various species, for example in cows its around 305 days, buffaloes- 275-300 days, goats - 114 to 187 days. For yak, its full lactation around 280 days (255-300 days), but in case it is not pregnant next year milking may be done which is called half lactation. In case of half lactation its around 150-180 days. Within this lactation period normal fluctuation is observed in total yield and its composition. If we divide the lactation period into three, in the 1st phase daily yield is increasing, then its reaches peak, then persistency and then declines. Live weigh, daily yield and dry matter intake of lactating animals is shown in the following figure graphically for easy understanding the relationship between three components.

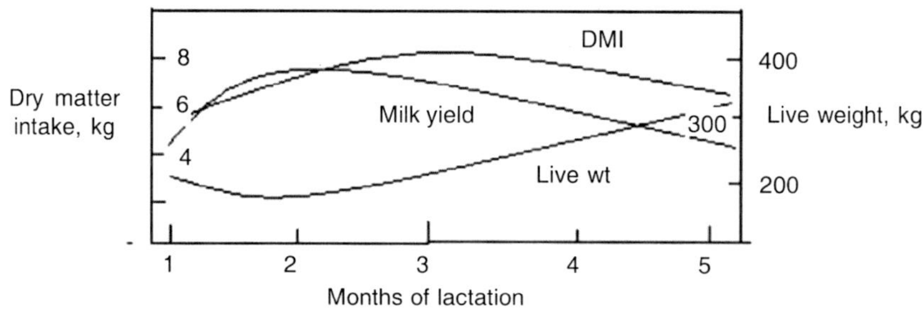

Table 7.12 : Milk composition of Tianzhu white yak of different stages of lactation.

	Early lactation (12 June)	Mid lactation (25 July)	Late lactation (20 Sept.)
Dry matter (percent)	16.1	17.8	16.3
SNF (percent)	10.9	12.3	10.5
Fat (percent)	5.1	5.4	5.8
Protein (percent)	5.2	5.7	4.7
Lactose (percent)	4.9	5.9	5.0
Ash (percent)	0.79	0.75	0.77
Energy (MJ/kg)	3.5	3.6	3.8

Zhang Rongchang *et al.*, (1986)

c. *Diurnal variation*: Percentage composition of milk as well as milk yield vary considerably from day to day. In general daily variation of milk yield are caused by excitement, estrus, incomplete milking and other irregularities previous milking to milking, disease, under feeding and related factors. Depression in milk yield that last for several days are usually accompanied by higher fat tests as because there is general inverse relationship between milk yield and fat tests. An incomplete milking fails to obtain the last drawn milk which is extremely high in fat. First drawn milk, on the other hand, is lowest in fat. Fat percent in morning and night milk may also vary perhaps due to relationship of pressure to milk and fat secretion, in which milk produced during long interval and against higher udder pressure which has a lower fat test and due to exercise which has a tendency to increase the level of milk fat. Consequently, the evening milk of animals at equal intervals produces milk that has slight higher fat content than does that obtained form morning milk.

d. *Parity and pregnancy*: Pregnancy has no apparent effect on fat content, rather SNF and protein increases with the advancement of pregnancy. Similarly, upto 6th or 7th year of age there is increase in milk yield thereafter declines.

e. *Exercise and disease*: Slight exercise apparently increased fat content without reducing the yield. Moderate to heavy exercise in high producing cows, however, will result in reduced milk secretion and a corresponding increase in fat content. Exercise has no apparent change in SNF content of milk. Any disease causes increase in body temperature frequently will be associated with increase in fat percent and decrease in SNF content. Udder infections like mastitis causes decline in milk fat, SNF, protein, lactose and a notable increase in the mineral and chloride contents of milk. Milk from mastitis is salty taste due to increased chloride contents. Ketosis reduces milk yield and subsequent increase fat content.

f. *Feeds and feeding*: Fat is the major composition which is affected by diet of the animals. Low roughage and/ or high concentrate/ grain diet, finely ground hay or green and lush pasture, pelleted feed and fish oil etc. depresses acetate production in rumen and subsequently the fat synthesis which decreases the fat content of milk. On the other hand, feeds especially high forage diet improves the fat content in milk. Changes in protein and SNF content of milk is less pronounced by environmental factors while minerals and lactose content are not all variable under normal farming situation. Trace minerals with the exception of Fe and Cu, can be increased by increasing in the diet upto certain limit. Fat soluble vitamins can be added through dietary manipulations and now a days, people are preparing functional foods rich in Se, Vitamin A, E etc. by adding in the diet. Though stability of these components needs to be evaluated from consumer health point of view. Ghosh *et al.* (2009) reported that an extra supplementation of Zn, Cu, Co and Mn in the ratio of 40:20: 2:1 to yak cows, milk production was significantly increased (126.58 g/d to 431.24g/d) and concluded that these trace mineral deficiency causes lowering of milk supplementation. Another most important factors influencing milk yield is pasture production - the quantity, growth status and nutritive value of the herbage. These are, in turn, affected by climate and season. All lactating yak, irrespective of age, parity or breed type and even location, tend to peak in yield in July and August when grass is at its best in terms of quality and quantity.

g. *Winter and cessation of milking*: As air temperature starts to fall after October and winter approaches rapidly, hand milking of the yak females is normally stopped. As indicated earlier, a yak does not dry off in consequence of this and continues to secrete a little milk for its calf. This happens irrespective of whether a female yak is pregnant or not. Only a cow that has lost her calf during the warm season will dry off when hand milking ceases. Similarly, a female that is pregnant but has been isolated from her previous calf will dry off when hand milking stops. Other pregnant females with a calf still at foot will not go dry until their one-year-old calf is removed prior to the next calving. Finally, a cow, even though not pregnant at the onset of winter but still suckling a calf, will continue to lactate through the following warm season and, normally, will be hand milked again. The half-lactating female yak (as it is called) will stop being milked at the end of her second warm season and will then go dry, irrespective of whether she is pregnant or not.

7.4.1 Milk production in a second year without calving again

Many yak do not conceive again in the year of calving. It is thus common in yak for lactation to continue into a second year. The amount of milk given over the months from December to May is very low, declining to perhaps as little as 2-4 litres in the whole of April. Yield then rises with the onset of grass growth and follows a monthly pattern similar to that already seen, but the amount produced in the second year is approximately half that given in the year of calving (sometimes up to two thirds and sometimes less); hence the name half-lactating commonly given to females milking into a second season without calving again - in contrast to the full-lactating yak in the year of calving. Parity differences are maintained in the second season at the lower level of yield. The fat percentage in the milk during the second half-lactating season is correspondingly higher than in the first full-lactating season, in line with the negative correlation between milk yield (quantity) and the fat percentage in the milk.

7.5 Factors influencing milk yield

Yak milk is dense and sweetish, with sweaty or yak hairy smell and greatly liked by the local people. The people who have not tasted may not like due to the peculiar smell, though its composition varies slightly among different yak breeds at different locations. Properties and composition of milk in different countries have already been discussed previously. Typically, the proportion of essential to nonessential amino acids is 0.8:1 as observed in a full analysis of amino acids in the milk of the Tianzhu White yak (Zhang Rongchang *et al.*, 1986) and 0.79:1, 0.67:1 and 0.72:1 in the milk of the Jiali, Pali and Sibu yak (Ji Qiumei, 2000a).

Table 7.13 : Milk yield of yak in various countries are not same and some of them are summarized below

Breed or yak of country	No.	Milk solid (percent)	Fat (percent)	Ash (percent)	Milk yield (kg ± SD)
Tianzhu White	17	16.9	5.5	0.77	141.7 ± 43.9
Jiulong	13	17.5	6.9	0.82	349.9 ± 131.9
Maiwa	24	17.5	6.3	0.82	176.5 ± 64.0
Jiali	21	16.3	6.8	0.95	104.5 ± 31.7
Pali	22	-	5.9	-	236.1 ± 74.9
Sibu	19	-	7.5	-	---
Kyrgyzstan	13	17.4	6.5	0.87	630
Nepal	12	17.4	6.5	0.90	---
India	14	17.9	6.5	0.87	238.4 ± 94.4

There are several factors which affect the milk yield in yak which may be again genetic or environmental. Some of the factors are discussed below.

a. *Species*: It is already discussed above how milk production varies from one species to another. Cattle, buffalo are producing more milk whereas sheep and goat are producing very less.

b. *Breed*: Among major factors, breed plays an important role as shown in the table 7.13, it is depicted that several breeds in the world are producing different quantities of milk, which is true to other milk producing breeds of cattle, buffalo, sheep and goat. Again, the crossbreds of local cows with yak bull gives more milk and for this purpose only farmers practicing the crossbreeding in the region, which one of major cause of declining yak population in yak rearing pockets.

c. *Persistency and stage of lactation*: There is considerable variation in the persistency of milk secretion and following peak production within 2 months of lactation. Individual yak shows very different persistency as some may show more milk production as compared to other during the peak yield. Some show sharp decline after peak yield and some may show slow decline i.e., good persistency. Milk production of the crossbreds is discussed later and they are having good persistency.

d. *Frequency of milking*: As yak are very poor milk producer, once or maximum twice milking is done.

e. *Pregnancy and parity*: Pregnancy reduces the milk production as compared to non-pregnant cows and its farmers' perception that upto 4th offspring, milk production increases and declines thereafter. Its true to cows also, where upto 5th or 6th calf its production increases and thereafter declines.

f. *Temperature and humidity*: Severe cold condition ceases milk production in yak and in very high temperature dry matter intake declines and thereby milk production decreased. During rainy season, in the higher elevations availability of pasture and meadows is greater and thereby increased milk production.

g. *Stress and disease*: Physical and physiological stress in animals negatively affect the milk production, similarly, diseases like infectious disease as well as metabolic diseases are adversely affected the milk production.

h. *Feeds and feeding* : Genetic potential for milk production of the animal is achieved only after nutritional requirements are made. The synthesis and diffusion of various milk constituents are dependant on presence and availability milk precursors in the blood. If precursors are available in sufficient quantity at proper ratio, then the process of milk synthesis is not hampered. In case when these are not met, then the milk secretion process limits to certain extent. Maintenance of lactation is closely related to adequate feed supply to the lactating animal. Dong *et al.* (2007) stressed that milking performance of yak should be improved by minimizing the negative effect of influencing factors through the following options:

i. Developing good yak breeds for dairy production or cross-breeds between yak and Simmental, Fresian, and Brown Swiss cattle.

ii. Improving native pastures through re-seeding, fertilization and introduction of fine grass species with high nutritive values.

iii. Supplementing lactating yaks with high quality forage, concentration and urea multi-nutrients blocks in harsh winter.

iv. Milking the cows once-a-day to keep calves and dams health.

v. Improving milking methods through training the milkman or machine-milking.

vi. Housing the milking females under the shed or in the pens on hot days to cool them down. The perspective of yak milk production is bright if all or most of these options are adopted timely and properly.

7.6 Fibre Production

Yak produce two types of fibre i.e., coarse outer hair and a fine down fibre, which grows prior to the onset of winter as additional protection for the yak against cold. The down fibre would be shed in early summer if not harvested. The down fibre may be used by the textile industry as an alternative to other fine animal fibres. Fabric made from yak down has better shine than wool and handles well. It provides a high degree of heat insulation. The income the herder receives from yak fibre is, at present, small relative to the income that can be obtained from yak milk and meat. None the less, the economic value of the down is leading to consideration of developing strains of yak with improved fibre production. Under field condition of Ladakh, even today aged man and women are seen to use hand made fabric from fibre along with the skin available from yak. The amount of fibre available from yak may be different depending on climate, and its association with breed, sex, age, season and method of harvesting the fibre from a particular animal. some of the predominant cause discussed below.

Breed, sex and location: As it is the protective cover of the animal, the higher dwelling breeds or animals living in higher elevations have the higher amount of fibre. Cai Li *et al.* (1980a) reported that highest amount of fibre may be obtained from Jiulong yak, especially selected for greater fibre production. Exceptional individuals of that breed are claimed to produce as much as 25 kg fibre, of which 50 percent is down fibre. This is ten-fold the yield of most ordinary yak. It is observed that the males have higher fibre production not only due to large body size but the females during lactation looses hair from the body. Steers also seen to loose its hair during drought in the summer months. Cai Li *et al.* (1987) reported that Jiulong breed of Sichuan province, fibre produced from males were 13.9 kg whereas from the female it was only 1.8 kg and from the steer it was 4.3 kg.

Method of harvesting: Combing out the down hair prior to shearing can increase the yield of down from the total fleece by about 10 percent compared with shearing alone. Wang Jie and Ouyang Xi, (1984) observed that the percentage of down fibre increased from about 50 percent with shearing to 61 percent with combing.

7.6.1 Fibres and staple properties

Like the other fibre wool, pashmina or hair yak fibre has its own properties which are summarized below.

Staple shape: This varies with the body part on which it grows and differs between the coarser hair and the down hair.

a. *Flat-topped type*- This is characteristic of down fibre of the best quality and is found especially in yak calves.

b. *Micro-braid type*- The fibres are even in thickness and relatively fine but less so, and longer, than the flat-topped type. This is found mostly in one-year-old yak.

c. *Sub-braid type*- The lower part of the staple is composed of down fibres and the upper part of mid-type and coarse hairs. This is seen often in the frontal parts of the body of one-year-old yak.

d. *Braid type*- The staple is composed largely of coarse hair and is typical of the hair on the yak's belly.

Fibre types: The fibres of the yak can be divided into three main types: down, mid-type and coarse.

a. *Down fibre*- Short, unmedullated fibres of less than 25 m in diameter, with irregular crimps and a soft luster.

b. *Mid-type hair*- Diameter between 25μ and 52.5μ. These hairs have a few large crimps. Some of the fibres have a latticed medulla. The hairs are longer than the down fibres and have a good luster.

c. *Coarse hair*- Diameter exceeds 52.5μ. The hairs have no crimps and are long. A proportion of them are medullated (18 percent according to Lu Zhonglin *et al.,* 1982). They have strong luster and poor textile quality.

Length and diameter of fibre: There are considerable differences in the length of stretched fibres, depending on the type of fibre and the part of the body. Zhang Rongchang (1989) reported that the length of coarse hair varying from 8.9 cm to 21.1 cm, and mid-type hair from 5.3 cm to 13 cm, with the longest in both cases on the belly and the shortest on the shoulder (and the fibres on the back intermediate in length). Diameter varies greatly with type of fibre and with breed and sex of animal, for any given fibre type there were no significant differences in the diameter of these fibres among the various body parts. Down fibres tend to be more uniform in diameter along their length than coarse hair fibres. In one study (Wang Jie and Ouyang Xi, 1984), the diameter was measured at the upper (outer end), middle and lower part of the fibre. Zhao Longquan *et al.,* (1994) observed the ratio, length and diameter of the different types of fibre on different parts of the body of 60 Plateau yak in Qinghai province depicted below in the table 7.14.

Table 7.14 : Measurements of different types of hair in different body parts.

Body part	Pro-portion	Coarse hair Length (cm)	Coarse hair Diameter (μ)	Prop-ortion	Mid-type hair Length (cm)	Mid-type hair Diameter (μ)	Prop-ortion	Down fibre Length (cm)	Down fibre Diameter (μ)
Shoulder	19.5	12.9	79.3	17.7	6.8	41.7	62.8	4.6	17.7
Back	21.1	13.3	81.0	15.0	8.8	39.2	63.9	4.6	16.6
Rump	20.4	17.9	84.9	18.9	9.6	39.8	60.7	4.2	17.5
Belly	63.6	19.0	86.7	29.5	10.2	39.0	6.9	3.8	16.7
Foreleg	60.3	19.3	88.6	33.9	10.1	43.4	5.7	3.8	18.4

Grease content: The lanolin content of yak hair is low. Lu Zhonglin *et al.* (1982) observed in grease content of male and female Gannan yak was 2.7 percent and 1.7 percent of the shorn fleece. Wang Jie and Ouyang Xi (1984) suggests that the grease content varies with the part of the body of the yak 3.8 percent on the back, 2.2 percent on the rump, 1.5 percent on the belly, and only 0.3 percent for hair from the tail.

7.7 Hides

Yak hide is a major source of raw hide in China - about one million yak hides are produced from the Qinghai-Tibetan Plateau per year. Under Indian condition, not much contribution has been seen from yak hide as the population is low enough. People of the high altitudes prefer to use this product for warm cloth prepared locally. Hide weight available from yak varies with breed or size of the breed as well as sex of the animal. it is observed that the weight of hide may vary from 14 kg in females to 35 kg in males. Zhang Rongchang (1989) reported that proportion weight of the hide to the live weight may vary from 5.5 in females to 8.8 percent in males. In Ladakh as well as in Arunachal Pradesh demand of hide is good and people prefers this for clothing but quality is often poorer than cattle hide.

7.7.1 Conservation of pure yak

There is a sharp decline of pure yak population in India especially due to indiscriminate breeding, mechanization in agriculture and transportation, shifting of occupation from animal husbandry to other activities and slow income generation from the sector for livelihood security and of course poaching of the animal at large numbers in higher altitudes. There is an urgent need to conserve the animal keeping view in mind its multipurpose activity adaptability in higher elevations.

There are several threats to this genetic resource (discussed below) which must be acknowledged and discussed to conserve the species with all stakeholders, though farmers thinking is that improvement of the breed / species means to make hybrid of yak with cows for higher productivity. So people should be aware about the conservation of the species by extension programmes.

- *Crossbreeding with exotic breeds*: Breeding programmes, by both governments and non-government organizations, have favoured the use of exotic breeds for crossbreeding, upgrading, or replacement. Although such programmes often fail to achieve their objectives (unless a stable supply of high inputs can be arranged) they have led to the dilution of indigenous breeds.
- *Agricultural intensification*: Changes in cropping patterns are a major factor leading to the elimination of indigenous farm animals. The switch to certain cash crops (such as tobacco) eliminates crop residues that used to be an important component of fodder. Adoption of hybrid wheat with its short stalks also reduces the availability of straw. Irrigation makes two or three crops a year possible, eliminating the possibility of grazing on stubble or browsing on trees in the fields.
- *Establishment of protected areas*: Wildlife sanctuaries, national parks and other types of protected areas almost always deprive livestock keepers of their pasture. Combined with efforts to persuade farmers to adopt high-input breeds, this contributes to the pressure on local breeds. Examples include the Kumbhalgarh Sanctuary in Rajasthan (which impinges on Nari cattle and Marwari camel) and the Grizzled Grey Squirrel Sanctuary in Tamil Nadu (which causes problems for the Malaimadu cattle breed) (Vivekanandan and Paulraj, 2002).
- *Lack of market demand*: Replacement of bullocks by tractors is a prime cause for the gradual extinction of draft animals.
- *Disappearance of traditional livelihoods*, coupled with loss of indigenous knowledge and institutions: making a living from keeping livestock is hard work that ties people down day in and day out. Many young people succumb to the attractions of city life. Animal-handling skills can disappear very quickly, within one generation. Village based breeding institutions, such as

keeping a community bull, also deteriorate rapidly once economic returns are not sufficient or social networks break down. Once such institutions have disappeared, they are very difficult to resurrect.

- Political conflicts and boundaries Warfare has contributed to the disappearance of indigenous breeds. Moreover, new boundaries, such as the Indo-Pakistan border, also disrupt migration patterns and undermine animal-dependent livelihood strategies. This has affected the Tharparkar breed (Köhler-Rollefson, 2000).

References

Bat-Erdene, T. (1993). Yield, composition and technological quality of yak milk. Uliastai Hot, Mongolia.

Cai Li *et al.* (1980a). [Agriculture and Livestock Bureau of Ganzi Tibetan Autonomous prefecture of Sichuan province and Southwest Nationalities College]. The good meat-purpose yak - the investigation and study of Jiulong Yak. Journal of China Yak, 1: 14-33.

Cai Li *et al.* (1984). [Yak Research Office of Southwest Nationalities College and Sichuan Grassland Institute] The research on the inter-specific cross combination between female yak and common bull. The research on the utilization and exploitation of grassland in the northwestern part of Sichuan province. National Publishing House of Sichuan province, Chengdu, China. pp. 107-113.

Cai Li *et al.* (eds) (1987). [Editorial Committee of Fauna of livestock and Poultry Breeds in Sichuan.] Fauna of Livestock and Poultry Breeds in Sichuan. Sichuan Science and Technology Publishing House, Chengdu, China.

Chen Xiafei *et al.* (1981). Investigation on Maiwa yak. Investigative reports on the resources of livestock and poultry breeds in Aba Tibetan Autonomous prefecture, Sichuan, China.

Chen Zhihua, Wen Yongli & Cai Li (1994). The systematic analysis of influence factors on the newborn weight of yak. Journal of Southwest Nationalities College (Natural Science Edition), 4: 325-331.

Dong S., Long, R., Kang, M. (2007). Milking performance of China yak (*Bos grunniens*): A preliminary report. African Journal of Agricultural Research 2(3): 52-57

Ghosh, M K and Bandopadhyay, S. (2007). Present nutritional status and future strategies for sustainable yak husbandry in India. Indian Farming. 56:3-8.

Ghosh, M K and Bandopadhyay, S. (2008). Effect of feeding regimes on growth performance and nutrient digestibility of Indian yaks under semi-intensive system. Indian Journal of Animal Sciences. 78: 117-119.

Ghosh, M.K., Konwar, P., Das, H.K., Bandopadhyay, S., Sasmal, D., Borah, B.K.D. and Bhattacharya. 2009. Effect of mineral supplementation on milk yield of yak. Proc. International Conference on yak husbandry- challenges and Strategies. NRC on Yak, ICAR.Dirang, Arunachal Pradesh.India.pp-92.

Ji Qiumei *et al.* (2000a). Analysis on milk output and milk quality of three good types of yak in Tibet. Journal of Gansu Agricultural University, 3: 269-276.

Ji Qiumei *et al.* (2000b). Analysis of producing flesh and flesh quality in three fine kinds groups yaks of Tibet. China Herbivore, 5: 3-6.

Ji Qiumei *et al.* (2000c). Research of yak produce performance in the Pali. China Herbivore, 6: 3-6.

Jialin, B. *et al.* (1998b). Meat production from crossbred and domestic yaks in China. Animal Science, 66: 465-469.

Joshi, D.D. (1982). Yak and Chauri Husbandry in Nepal. H.M. Kathmandu, Government Press, Singha Durbar. XVII, 145 pp.

Kandeepan, G, Sangma, S, Paul, V and Jaykumar, S. 2010. Quality charavteristics of low fat paneer developed from yak milk. Indian Journal of Animal Sciences. 80: 932-33.

Kataktalware, M A, Pourouchottamane, R, Rajkhowa, J, Barua, K, Borah, S, Sarkar, M, and Bhattacharya, M. 2007. Effect of castration on pack performance of yak. Indian-Veterinary-Journal. 84: 1173-1175

Köhler-Rollefson, I. 2000. *Management of animal genetic diversity at community level.* Managing Agrobiodiversity in Rural Areas, GTZ, Eschborn, Germany.

Lang Jie, Zhou Daorong & Wu Xianzhi (1999). Report on the breeding by milk ability of Maiwa yak. Journal of Sichuan Grassland, 4: 50-53.

Lei Huanzhang *et al.* (1983). Report on the investigation of yak in Qinghai. Investigative report on the resource of livestock and poultry breeds in Qinghai province. pp. 50-101.

Lei Huanzhang *et al.* (1985). Studies on the ecological reaction of criss-cross grazing of yak and its hybrid in the cold and warm seasons. Journal of China Yak, 2: 13-23.

Li Quan *et al.* (2000b). Measurement of milk performance in domestic yak in Guoluo Prefecture. Chinese Journal of Animal and Veterinary Sciences, 3: 10-11.

Liu Haibo (1989). China Yakology. Sichuan Science and Technology Publishing House, Chengdu, China. pp. 119-123.

Lu Zhonglin *et al.* (1982). The hair quantity of Luqu yak. Journal of Southwest Nationalities College (Animal Husbandry and Veterinary Sciences Edition), 1: 17-20.

Luo, X L, Tong, Wei, Z B, Xin, Y, P and Zhao, Q. 2006. Meat characteristics of Qinghai yak and semi-wild yak, Animal Science Journal. 77: 230-34

Ma Zongxiang & Dou Yaozong (1982). Study on the growth pattern in terms of seasonal body weight change. Journal of China Yak, 4(1): 21-28.

Mondal, D and Pal, R N. 1996. Chemical composition of yak milk. Indian Journal of Dairy Science. 49(6). 413-414

Pourouchottamane, R, Chatterjee, A, Kataktalware, MA, Saravanan, BC, and Sarkar, M. 2007. Growth performance of male yak calves fed on different levels of concentrate. Indian Veterinary Journal. 2007. 84: 1156-1158

Pu Ruitang *et al.* (1987). Determination on the meat composition and meat performance of Tianzhu White yak. Journal of China Yak, 4: 22-25.

Sarmah, DK, Raquib, M, Ghosh, K and Bhattacharya,M 2009. Standardization of low fat milk dahi based on organoleptic attributes. Proc. International Seminar on Yak Husbandry- Challenges and strategies. NRC on Yak, ICAR,Dirang, Arunachal Pradsh. India.pp-167-168.

Smirnov, D A, Shevkhuzhev, A F, Gusel'nikova, A A and Kokurina, T, M. 1990. Meat yield and meat quality of yaks. Doklady-Vsesoyuznoi-Ordena-Lenina-i-Ordena-Trudovogo-Krasnogo-Znameni-Akademii-Sel'-skokhozyaistvennykh-Nauk-im-VI-Lenina. 1: 46-49. CABI abstract.

Vivekanandan, P. and B. Paulraj. 2002. "Community conservation of 'Malai Madu' breed of cattle". pp. 81–90 in: LPPS. *Local livestock breeds for sustainable rural livelihoods: Towards community-based approaches for animal genetic resource conservation*. Proceedings of a conference/workshop held on 1–4 November, 2000 in Udaipur and Sadri, Rajasthan, India. Lokhit Pashu-Palak Sansthan, Sadri, India.

Wang Jie & Quyang Xi, (1984). Physical features of yak hair. Journal of Southwest Nationalities College (Animal Husbandry and Veterinary Sciences Edition), 1: 25-29.

Wei Ronglu *et al.* (1981). Analyses of effect on meat of F1 hybrid of inter-specific cross between female yak and common bull. Journal of China Yak, 2: 5-15.

Wen Yongli *et al.* (1993). Influences of two simple methods of supplement during the winter on the performances of female yaks. Journal of Southwest Nationalities College (Natural Science Edition), 19: 236-241.

Zang Yinsong (1985). Observation and analysis on milk production of yak in Qilian area. Journal of China Yak, 1: 51-56.

Zhang Rongchang (1989). China: the yak. Gansu Scientific and Technology Press, Lanzhou, China. 386 pp.

Zhang Rongchang *et al.* (1986). Determination on the main composition in milk of Tianzhu White yak. Journal of China Yak, 2: 23-26.

Zhao Longquan *et al.* (1994). Hair and down hair analysis of yak of Plateau type in Qinghai Province. Journal of Qinghai Animal Husbandry and Veterinary Medicine, 2: 29-31.

Zhong Guanghui *et al.* (1996). Correlation analysis between body formation traits and heart girth in Jiulong yak. Journal of Southwest Nationalities College (Natural Science Edition), 4: 409-413.

Zi, X D, Zhong, G H, Wen, Y L, Zhong J C, Liu, C L, Ni,Y A, Yezi, Y H and Ashi,M G. 2004. Growth performance, carcass composition and meat quality of jiulong-yak (*Bos grunnien*). Asian Australian Journal of Animal Sciences. 17:410-414.

❑❑❑

Chapter 8

Hybridization and Performance of Hybrids

8.1 Introduction

Hybridization may be defined as the planned mating of unrelated individuals for better progeny. This is tool for improvement of animals since new genes can not be created, though they can recombine into more desirable groupings. Research and development aimed at bringing the genetic improvement of domestic yak, will have to be planned keeping the view of the uniqueness of the species, its multiple use in human civilization at very high altitude, but in this chapter we will discuss the mating of yak with low producing desi or crossbred cows to improved production in terms of milk, meat and drought power. Since, the yak belongs to bovidae family it can bred with cattle. In fact, species hybridization of domestic yak and hill cattle, zabu or exotic cattle is common practice in yak rearing places. In china, yellow cattle (*Bos taurus*), zebu cattle are also bred to yak male since time immemorial. Low conception rate of hybrids produced from yak and other cattle breeds, crossbreeding between yaks and cattle is limited to only the F_1 and F_2 generations. The F_3 generation (containing about 12.5% yak gene have difficulty surviving at high-altitude (above 3000 m) in

Qinghai-Tibet Plateau and therefore, F3 hybrids are seldom produced. Since, artificial insemination is inevitably restricted to more accessible areas and maintenance of improved breeds is difficult and expensive, most crossbreeding programs use locally available cattle. Under Indian condition, especially in Ladakh, yaks are hybridized upto 4th generation for better productivity and perception is that when cattle gene comes down to 6.25 percent (4th generation) it resembles yak and need not to further bred for any purposes.

8.2 Purpose of hybridization

1. The purpose of any crossbreeding or hybridization is to introduce some good trait to the F_1 or successive generation and if it happens the term called heterosis or hybrid vigour. In the case of hybrids of yak with *Bos taurus* or *Bos indicus* cattle, the males always sterile and females are fertile. Successive breeding with hybrid females with yak will have some advantages and disadvantages. In general, the hybrids occupy a different niche from that of the pure yak in the economy of the pastoral mountain regions, mostly at the lower elevations. Part of the explanation for this may arise from a less well developed physiological adaptation of the hybrids to high altitude, for example in terms of their pulmonary haemo-circulatory adaptations. Therefore, adaptability and productivity of the hybrid yak get severely affected at very high altitude.

2. Interspecies hybrids also offer clues in the search for answers to several other questions of genetics and gene expression including overdominance, hybrid vigor, inbreeding depression, and segregation distortion.

3. Hybridization is often done early in the breeding season with yak cows at their first oestrus (between June and September), so that, hybrid animals are born March to July than are the pure yak and if not conceived may be kept for artificial insemination from exotic bull's semen. But in terms of comparing the performance of hybrids with that of yak or cattle it introduces a further complication. Date of birth affects the subsequent performance of the animals because they have a better start before the following winter. Such an advantage can be seen over the first two years of life, and possibly longer. Nevertheless, the comparisons of the performance of hybrids with that of yak and, where possible, cattle are highly suggestive of a part played by

heterosis. This arises because the performance is not only better than that of the yak when kept alongside them but also, in some cases, better than that of the local hilly cattle as most of the cases these are very less productive. Therefore, the presumption is that purebred females of the improved breeds would yield effectively nothing if kept like typical yak. Jingfu *et al.* (2000) studied the growth of F1 generation from (Simmental × local yellow cattle) × yak and (Holstein × local yellow cattle) × yak (group 1 was (Simmental ×local yellow cattle) × yak, in which male hybrid of Simmental × local yellow cattle was introduced from Linxia County; group 2 was (Holstein × local yellow cattle) × yak, male hybrid of Holstein × local yellow cattle introduced from Linxia County; group 3 was (Simmental × local yellow cattle) × yak, male hybrid of Simmental × local yellow cattle introduced from Jinchuan County, and group 1, group 2, group 3 were experimental groups; group 4 was yak × yak, came from local yak was the control group) and concluded that

a) Hybrids of Simmental × local yellow cattle naturally mating with yak and Holstein × local yellow cattle naturally mating yak, of which hybrid of Simmental × local yellow cattle and Holstein × local yellow cattle introduced from Jinchuan and Linxia County, had heavy weight, rapid growth, high survival rate and obvious heterosis.

b) Body measurement and body weight of group were smaller than those of group 1 and group 2. The reason that there is something to do with heredity and other factors in different introduced areas.

c) According to thesis of phenotypic value of production performance, the phenotypic value is the effected result by heredity and environment, and fine breed must need good feeding, introduced local yellow cattle hybrids, matching female yak and F1 generation must strengthen feeding and management. Practice half-cowshed feeding in the cold seasons and graze in warm seasons, added with complementary feeds. And practice full milking for calves; thus, hybrids had better heterosis, and could get better economy benefit.

8.3 Nomenclature of the various progenies

In Ladakh, various progenies have different name shown in the table 8.1 and in different places of yak rearing countries have their own names.

Table 8.1 : Nomenclature of different progenies in local language of Ladakh

Progeny	Male	Female
F_1	*Tzo* (pronounce as jo)	*Tzomo* (pronounce as jomo)
F_2	*Tor*	*Tormo*
F_3	*Gar*	*Garmo*
F_4	*Tde* (pronounce as dee)	*Tdemo* (pronounce as deemo)

8.4 Production Performance of Hybrids

Purpose of interspecies hybridization is to improve the productivity of the next generation, so that their utility remains viable at the very high altitude. The performances of the hybrid yak varies considerably depending upon the breed of cattle used and area where the hybrid animals are kept. Chinese workers reported that the birth weight of hybrids produced by mating yak females and local Chinese (yellow cattle) bulls could be as much as 50% heavier than pure yak calves (Zhao, 1984). Reports from other countries also suggest a substantial increase in birth weight of hybrids resulting from crosses of yak females and males of a local breed of cattle (e.g. increases of about 15% and 30 - 40% for Buryatia (Katzina *et al.,* 1994) and Mongolia (Zagdsuren, 1994), respectively), with the extent of the increase dependent upon the types of yak, breeds of local cattle used, and husbandry practices. Although hybridization is very common under Indian condition for the better productivity in terms of milk, meat and wool, but relevant data are not available due the absence of systematic study in this direction.

8.4.1 Growth

The simplest manifestation of growth in farm animals is their increased in size and weight. All animals start their lives as single cell weighing practically nothing, then grow to reach mature body weight that ranges from 10 kg for yak calf to almost 300 kg or more at adult stage. The pattern by which animals grow from conception to maturity can be represented by a sigmoid curve (S shaped), which shows upto certain period growth accelerates and after that it decelerates and then very low. The growth of a particular animal depends upon the physical environment, supply of nutrients and prevalence of disease surrounding the animal. In general, animals reared under intensive system will follow the sigmoid curve and will be different from extensive system of management. At the same, time location of the animal is also important as hybrid in lower altitudes grow faster than the animals of higher altitudes which may be attributed by adaptation characteristics. Nutrition of the dam during pregnancy or body condition of the dam is also important factor for growth of the offspring. In addition to these factors, season of calving plays an important role in birth weight and survivability of the offspring as it is again related to nutrient availability to the dam as well as calves. Zhao Bingyao *et al.* (1984) and Zhang Jiachuan (1984) studied the effect of dam weight, altitude and environment on birth weight of calves and did not find any impact. Cai Li (1989) reported that the F_1 yak hybrids from Holstein-Friesian bulls were the heaviest and largest, followed by the hybrids from yak mated to bulls of yellow cattle. The backcrosses were smaller than the F_1. The backcrosses to yellow cattle bulls were actually smaller than the local yak, which suggests that the cattle involved in the hybridization may have been very small indeed - but in the absence of this information, this is speculation (table 8.2).

Table 8.2 : Body weight and various body measurements of various yak crossbred

Type of animal	Sex	No.	Adult weight (kg)	Height at withers (cm)	Body length (cm)	Heart girth (cm)	Cannon bone circumference (cm)
Local yak	F	73	249	118.3	138.1	160.3	16.9
	S	12	443	128.7	161.5	198.0	20.6
Yak (F) × HF*(M)	F	42	357	121.8	125.3	182.7	18.5
("improved" F1)	S	7	580	144.0	178.3	215.6	21.3
Yak (F) × yellow	F	47	292	118.3	148.0	167.9	17.0
cattle (M) (local F1)	S	14	477	128.7	173.0	197.3	20.3
F1 (F) × HF*cattle	F	19	262	116.4	136.6	165.6	18.1
(M) ("improved"B1)	S	6	521	150.0	174.5	206.5	22.5
F1 (F) × yellow cattle or yak (M) (local B1)	F	10	177	100.5	118.9	146.1	14.1

Note: F= female; S = steer (castrated male); M=male; HF* = Holstein-Friesian or (75 % HF + 25 % yellow cattle).

Cai Li (1989)

Body weight and linear body dimensions of adult Maiwa yak F1 hybrids from Maiwa yak females mated to bulls of yellow cattle or Holstein-Friesian (or 75 % HF + 25 % yellow cattle) and backcrosses involving these types -in Hongyuan, Ruoergai and Ganzi counties of Sichuan.

Like the yak, hybrids of yak with cattle show similar responses to the seasonal cycles of grass growth, with rapid growth during the warm season followed by severe loss over the winter and recovery the following year (Xiao Zhiqing, 1984).

8.4.2 Meat production

Meat production is the result of growth performance of the animal. If the growth of an animal is faster enough, the meat quantity from that particular animal will be higher in a particular period. The rule is same for yak also and the factors promote growth will enhance the meat production. A number of studies have also examined the meat output, at slaughter, of hybrids of yak derived from mating of yak with both local cattle and the different exotic breeds (Cai Li, 1989). Numbers in the breed groups examined tend to be small and there are no consistent differences between the breeds of sire in dressing percentage or the yield of meat. Nor do these differ from pure yak. There are differences in carcass weight, but only in so far as this is related to slaughter weight. Of the animals described in the above table (table 8.1) that were slaughtered at 17 months old, it was found that the hybrids had reached slaughter weights around 50 percent greater than the yak at the same age. Thus, the hybrids provided a proportionately much greater yield of meat from the carcass than yak at that age. Katzina *et al.* (1994) also reported slaughter weights of hybrid animals at 18 - 20 months old that were 25 - 30 percent heavier than for yak at that age in the Buryatia region of Russia. They reported further big increases in the growth of the hybrid if slaughter was delayed for another year. Under Indian condition, animals above 5 years of age is being slaughtered and only during the months winter. In Ladakh, road remain close after heavy snow fall from the month of November to April. Availability of essential food items is scarce for local people. People mostly depends upon th meat from the locally available animals like sheep, goat etc. Like other meat animals, yak are slaughter for meat especially during the winter season when food scarcity is severe for human as well as for the animals.

Supplementary feeding of concentrates during the winter, have both been shown to give a marked response in weight gain (Langjie Zeren *et al.*, 1987) and in the proportion of meat in the carcass of hybrids of yak with, for example, the Holstein-Friesian (Li Xuewen *et al.*, 1983). Under our situation, hardly any animals especially yak supplemented for growth or meat purpose, rather fed only agricultural by products or roughages.

8.4.3 Milk production

Since time immemorial crossbreeding is going on to get some desirable trait in the offspring. Hybridizing the yak with cattle is to get the farmer with additional milk for their own use or for sale. The larger quantity of milk made available is a consequence of the higher yield from such hybrids relative to the yak but also because all or most of the milk from the F_1 is taken by the herdsmen. Lactation period of the pure yak varies from 250- 280 days (Mondal, 2010), though farmers reported that it goes upto 200 days in most of the cases and then left for high hill grazing. In case of crossbreds (*Tzomo*) lactation period is around 300 days under intensive system of management the yield of milk for the whole lactation period around 750-800 kg with the maximum yield 4.05 kg per day provided the animal is supplemented with concentrate and mineral mixture. In pure yak fat percent in milk is around 10 percent, whereas in the crossbreds, it decreased to around 6-7 percent. Some of the studies with milk production performance is presented below for better understanding.

Table 8.3 : Daily milk yield and fat percentage for different types of F_1 hybrids

Type of animal	Daily milk yield (kg)	Fat (%)
Local yak	2.0	6.3
Yak (F) × Holstein-Friesian (M) ("improved" F1)	8.0	5.4
Yak (F) × local (yellow) cattle (M) (local F1)	3.0	6.0
F1 (F) × Holstein-Friesian cattle (M) ("improved" B)	5.5	
F1 (F) × local (yellow) cattle (M) (local B1)	0.5-1.0	6.2

B = backcross, F = female, M = male
(Cai Li, 1989)

The F_1 hybrids from the predominantly Holstein-Friesian bulls are seen (table 8.4) to have yielded a much higher daily amount of milk than the yak (Xu Guiling *et al.*, 1983). But the backcrosses in this case have regressed in yield, as would be expected if the initial F1 advantage is partly attributable to hybrid vigour. In the case of the ordinary F1 hybrid (F1 involving local cattle), the yield is higher than that of the pure yak, but the backcrosses, perhaps surprisingly, gave less milk per day than the yak cows. However, no milk yields are reported for the local cattle, which, as in comparable results of Joshi (1982) from Nepal, may have had lower milk yields than the yak.

Table 8.4 : Milk yield in different types of F1 hybrid

Yak female mated to:	Age (year)	Parity	No.	Milk yield mean (kg) for 150 days	Fat (%)
HF	3	1	26	689	5.3
HF	4	1	15	809	5.2
HF	4	2	3	919	5.2
HF (half lactation)*	4	1	4	494	6.5
Various**	3	1	7	576	4.9
Yak	4	1	6	226	7.3

HF= Holstein-Friesian or crosses of HF with local cattle breeds
* half- lactation" - a second lactation in the year following first calving without a further pregnancy,
** various breeds of exotic cattle sire used
Xu Guiling *et al.*, 1983

It is also of interest from the results of above mentioned table that the hybrids, like the yak, have the capacity to give milk in a second year without another intervening pregnancy - although, again as in the yak - the yield in the second year is reduced relative to that in the first. Though, Jain and Yadava (1985) present results from F_1 hybrids of yak with hill zebu bulls in Himachal Pradesh which suggest that the daily milk yield of the hybrids was only half-way between that of the parent species (no heterosis) - but again no information is given on whether the three types of animals (ten animals in each group) were treated alike. It is quite possible that they were not, as all the animals were not from the same place. Surprisingly, the milk from this F1 hybrid is reported as having had a significantly higher fat content

(7.32 percent) than that of the yak (6.45 percent) (in spite of a higher daily milk yield in the hybrid) and much higher fat percentage than that of the hill zebu cows (4.17 percent). This result is difficult to explain and at variance with other investigations. Wen Yongli *et al.* (1987) observed that the supplementary feeding of hybrids of yak and the Holstein-Friesian with urea, minerals and some ground corn during the warm grazing season led to an increase in milk yield of 10 percent in full-lactating animals (those that had calved that year) and 20 percent in "half-lactating" cows (those that had last calved in the previous year). The workers also remarked that this will benefit the farmer economically. Moreover, the availability of supplementary feed in winter would be severely restricted in practice to localities where pastures have been improved and where agricultural products are also available. Not only milk yield, but milk let down also be affected by hybridization as Zhang Rongchang *et al.* (1983) observed that milk came out of the udder about 50 percent more quickly than from the yak cows and the pressure required to extract the milk was lower.

8.4.4 Draught and work performance

Yak is an useful animal in the high altitudes as these can carry heavier loads than other animals (around 150 kg) and F_1 hybrids of yak females mated to bulls of local cattle, and the reciprocal hybrids, are widely used for draught - both for ploughing and as pack animals. The hybrids are easily tamed and appear to have better heat tolerance than pure yak, which make them very suitable for work even comparatively at low altitude. The hybrids produced from mating yak bulls to local female cattle are used mainly for ploughing. Liu Qigui (1981) showed that with a traditional-style plough, two ordinary F1 hybrid steers making a furrow 15 cm wide can till around 0.13 ha per day. With a more modern plough (producing a 24.8 cm-wide furrow), two mature hybrid steers in medium fat condition ploughed 605 sq m in one hour on moderately moist, flat ground. Per unit body weight, the maximum draught power of mature hybrid steers in reasonably good condition has been measured as exceeding that of the pure yak. The authors also reported that respiration and pulse rates of the animals returned to normal in less than half an hour after completion of ploughing. Reports about the performance of the F1 hybrid as a pack animal on grassland, the F_1 hybrid has been found to carry 75 kg, equal to 16.3 percent of its body weight, and to cover 30 km in six hours. The respiration and pulse rates had returned to normal in 53 minutes after reaching to its destination.

Table 8.5 : Carrying capacity of yak steer and F_1 hybrid steer

Breed	No.	Age (years)	Live weight (kg)	Load (kg)	Load/ live weight (%)	Distance (km)	Time (hr)	Recovery time (min)
Yak steer	4	6 - 11	408.1	75	18.4	30	7.2	50.0
F1 steer	3	10 - 14	459.6	75	16.3	30	6.0	53.3

Zhang Rongchang, (1989)

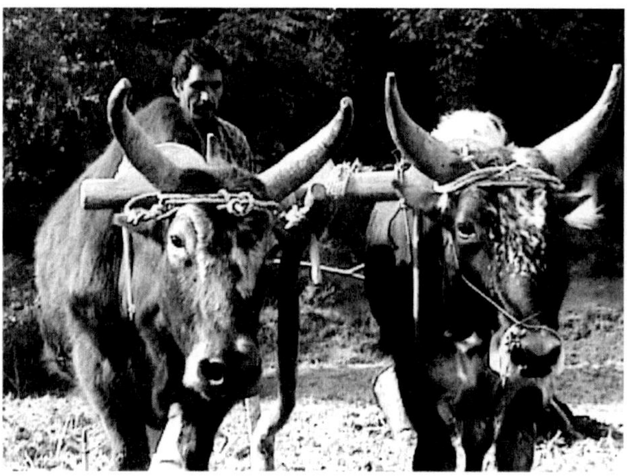

Crossbred Yak in Agricultural Operation

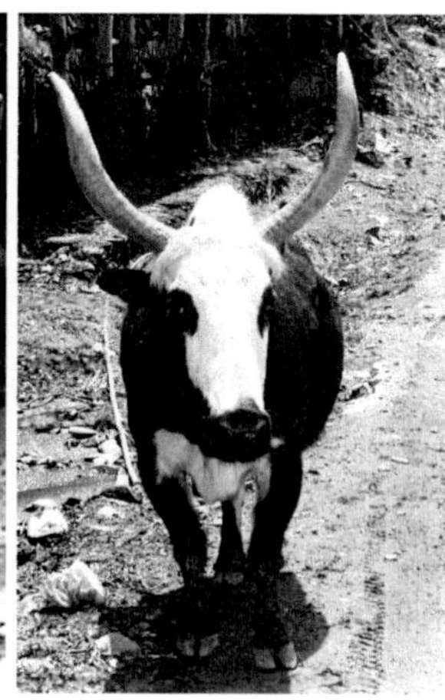

Crossbred Yak

8.5 Reproduction and fertility

Female hybrids, first-cross and backcross generations, have normal fertility. Males, however, are sterile until there have been several generations of backcrossing (to either yak or common cattle).

8.5.1 Female Reproduction

Estrus

Estrus in the F1 hybrids is seasonal and affected by climate and nutrition as seen in yak, but the hybrids attains puberty approximately 1 year earlier than yak. Therefore, F1 hybrid females are usually mated at 25 - 28 months of age and they calve for the first time at about 3 years of age. Estrus can occur several times during the breeding season if the crossbred female has not been mated or not conceived successfully. Signs of estrus in the F_1 female are more obvious than in the pure yak i.e., normally developed follicles, a proportion slightly higher than in contemporary yak, reddish vaginal membrane, mild discharge from vagina and more importantly mounting to other animals.

Gestation Length

Average gestation length of hybrids is same to the cattle and farmers under Indian condition reported that this is not affected by any other factors and generation. Cai Li (1989) reported that the gestation length in crosses of yak with ordinary local cattle as 278 days whereas Denisov (1938) reported an average gestation length of 282 days for F_1 females mated back to Schwyz cattle bulls and 265 days for those mated back to yak bulls.

Survival of calves

Survival of the offsprings to the age of six months is very similar in F_1 hybrids and first backcrosses to that of pure yak. Thus, relative to the yak, the F_1 hybrid has a better overall reproductive rate over a lifetime. The equally good survival of the first backcross (B_1) is observed by Cai Li (1989). This viewpoint, however, has to be seen in the context that herdsmen generally wish to keep as much milk as possible from the F_1 dams for their own use or for sale. Farmers perception is that the survival of the hybrids are depends mostly the elevation/location and management system of the herd, rather genetic one as hybrid perform better in lower altitudes with concentrate and mineral supplementation. At the same time they opined that season of breeding/ calving, nutritional status of the dam and supplementary feeding to dam as well as newborn have an impact on the overall survival rate of the hybrids.

Abortion and dystocia

Difficulty in normal parturition process is called as dystocia which may be genetic, anatomical or pathological. Due to genetic differences between yaks and other cattle breeds, there are placental abnormalities that may result in inadequate support of fetal development. Abortion occurs more frequently when yaks carry a hybrid foetus. In a survey of 5623 matings (to produce hybrids) in Hongyuan County, Sichuan, from 1976 to 1982, the abortion rate was 20.7% (Zhang, 1989). Although the causes of abortion have not been established, it is speculated that genetic differences, placental underdevelopment and environmental conditions such as cold weather and low oxygen content of the air may be involved. Dystocia is more common with hybrid fetuses than yak fetuses. A survey from Hongyuan County in 1979 showed that of 1144 calvings, 32.8% required assistance (5% were delivered by laparotomy). Therefore, it is recommended that large females have to be used to produce hybrid calves.

8.5.2 Male reproduction

As discussed earlier, the male offspring of the yak crosses are always sterile. The external genitalia, libido, and mating behavior of the crossbred male are normal but there are no sperm in the seminal fluid. Therefore, the crossbred behave like a natural teaser bull. First and second backcross generations are also sterile. By the third generation of backcross (15/16 yak or cattle blood) some spermatocytes are usually present and the occasional male is fertile. Fertility is not assured until the fourth or fifth generation of backcross (Zhong, 1994). In practice, however, intact males of the backcross generations are rarely seen, since there is no good reason to produce them. Therefore, precise data on the proportions of bulls showing normal spermatogenesis in successive generations of backcrossing are not available. It is well established that there are no spermatogonia in the seminiferous tubules of F1 and early generations of backcrosses. Possible causes for this have been considered in the structure of the X and Y chromosomes; these structures differ in certain respects among crosses, pure yak and pure cattle (Gao *et al.*, 1983). In particular, the arm ratios differ, most notably for the Y-chromosomes. There are differences among hybrids, yak and ordinary cattle in the proportions of different cell types in the anterior pituitary gland, resulting in reduced production of follicle stimulating hormone (FSH) in hybrids. However, frequent injection of FSH and leutinizing hormone (LH) intravenously in well-fed crossbred calves increased libido but did not result in sperm production at 12 months of age (Cai and Weiner, 1995).

References

Cai Li. Wiener G. 1995. *The Yak*. Regional Office for Asia and the Pacific of the Food and Agriculture Organization of the United Nations, Bangkok, Thailand. 111-114.

Cai Li. 1989. *Sichuan yak*. Chengdu, China, Sichuan Nationality Press. 223 pp.

Denisov VF. 1938. Hybridization of the yak with Kirghiz cattle and the Schwyz. *CAB Animal Breeding Abstracts*. 7:116-117.

Gao AP, Huang WX. 1983. A study on the chromosomes of yak, common cattle and their hybrid. In: *Hengduan Mountain in Research of Qinghai-Tibet Plateau*. Yuannan People's Publishing House. 365-372.

Jingfu, G. Jiang Shihai and Luo Guangrong, 2000. Growth measurements of F1 generation from yak with ordinary cattle. *Proc. Yak Production In Centralasian Highlands*.

Jain, Y.C. & Yadava, R.S. 1985. Yield and composition of milk of Himachali yak, yak hybrid and hill come. *Indian Journal of Animal Sciences*, 55: 223-224.

Joshi, D.D. 1982. *Yak and chauri husbandry in Nepal*. H.M. Kathmandu, Government Press, Singha Durbar. 145 pp.

Katzina, E.V., Davydov, V.N. & Baldanov, N.D. 1994. Elaboration of the scheme of production and usage of industrial hybrids of yak and meat cattle. Proceedings of the first international congress on yak. *Journal of Gansu Agricultural University* (Special issue June 1994) pp. 44-48.

Langjie Zeren *et al.* 1987. Supplementary feeding trial for fattening hybrids of Holstein Friesian x yak in warm season. *Journal of China Yak*, 4: 51-55.

Li Xuewen, *et al.* 1983. The preliminary test of hybrid's fattening and slaughtering. *Journal of China Yak*, 1: 35-37.

Liu Qigui. 1981. Report of investigation of Hongyuan yak in Sichuan. *Journal of China Yak*, 3: 69.

Mondal, G. 2010. Yak husbandry: An overview. *Agro- Animal Resources of Higher Himalayas*. Eds. D.H Dwivedi, S.K. Dwivedi and S. Gupta. Satish Serial Publishing House. New Delhi. Chapter 17. pp- 385-401.

Wen Yongli, Wu Kang & Zhang Zhongming.1987. The study on improving milk production of female F1 hybrid with supplementary feeding in warm season in the frigid pastoral area. *Journal of Southwest Nationalities College* (Animal Husbandry and Veterinary Sciences Edition), 2: 44-47.

Xiao Zhiqing. 1984. Preliminary evaluation of growth and development of F1 hybrid from different sires. *Journal of Southwest Nationalities College* (Animal Husbandry and Veterinary Sciences Edition), 2: 17-22.

Xu Guiling, Wang Gensheng, & Shi Aijuan. 1983. Analysis of factors related with the milking performance and milk quality of yak. *Journal of China Yak*, 1: 21-29.

Zagdsuren, Yo. (1994). Heterosis in yak hybrids. Proceedings of the first international congress on yak. *Journal of Gansu Agricultural University* (Special issue, June 1994) pp. 59-62.

Zhang Jiachuan. 1984. The test of cross combination of yak and cattle. *Journal of South-west Nationalities College* (Animal Husbandry and Veterinary Sciences Edition), 1: 30-35.

Zhang Rongchang, Kong Linglu and Jin Yong. 1983. The milking characteristics of yak and chauri. *Journal of China Yak*. 1: 14.

Zhang YC. 1989. *China: The Yak*. Lanzhou, Gansu, China: Gansu Science and Technology Press. 219-226.

Zhao Bingyao *et al*. 1984. An experiment on the cross combination of interspecific hybridization between female yak and cattle bull. *Journal of Chin Yak*, 1: 47-70.

Zhao BY. 1984. An experiment on the cross combination of interspecies hybridization between female yak and common bull. *J China Yak*. 1:47-50.

Zhong Jingcheng. 1994. Polygenic inheritance unbalance hypothesis about sterility of the male yak-cattle (hybrid). Proceedings of the first international congress on yak. *Journal of Gansu Agricultural University* (Special issue June 1994) pp. 284-287.

Chapter 9

Behaviour

The way in which an organism, or group responds to a certain set of conditions is known as behaviour. Animal behaviour not only studies what animals do, but also how, why, where and when they do it. Behavior is a predictable thing. Behaviour studies have played an important role for better understanding of the animals. People have probably always been fascinated by the behavior of animals. Indeed an understanding of the behavior of prey animals must have been essential to our early ancestors; their paintings on the walls of caves suggest that they could have been fairly familiar with behavioral concepts such as herd size and migration.

Behaviourally, the yak is active and easily excited and can have a ferocious temper. Its conditioned reflexes make it respond rapidly to danger and external forces. In the grazing situation, yak will often jump and run, pursuing each other with tail in the air. Yak can gallop like a horse - an attribute that is enjoyed by herdsmen who organize annual races. Yak can also roll over on pastures as horses do - but unlike other bovines. The yak is extremely nimble in its mountainous terrain despite its impressive size, and is so well adapted to colder climates that it would not survive in milder conditions. Yak have the ability to be readily trained. This ability helps the herdsmen in the feeding and management of the yak, especially as most yak graze year round and are not housed and not usually fenced in or tethered, except for milking. The yak are trained by the herdsmen to return to the campsite by the call of their names, or by special cries or singing. Yak are also readily tamed and trained for use as pack animals or for riding. Once trained, yak retain their acquired behaviour.

The yak have evolved specialized adaptations to thrive at the cold high altitudes. To deal with lower oxygen tension at a very high altitude, they posses an extra pair of ribs resulting in a larger lung capacity. To deal effectively with the cold, they have a long luxurious coat consisting of an inner jacket of warm, soft down and long soft outer hair plus a dense undercarriage of long hair that hangs down from the belly sometimes touching the ground. To adapt in the region where feed scarcity is severe, they have a smaller rumen than do other cattle breeds and this produces a slower outflow of materials through the digestive tract. The longer residence time of feed in the digestive system is partially responsible for the yak's ability to thrive on lower quality forage and indirectly a lower food consumption. They tend to put on a healthy layer of fat near the skin from spring through autumn when graze is plentiful and then eat less in the winter, when there is hardly any feed available for the animals. This fat layer in addition to providing energy reserves for the winter, acts as thermal insulation to conserve body heat, a survival adaptation in contrast to heat generating mechanisms. They prefer to stay out of the wind during the coldest days or will face into the wind as their long thick forehead and front quarter hair is thicker there than on the backside.

Yak has exceptional stamina and agility, and can climb well. They are grazer as well as browser. Females and young congregate in large herds, while adult males spend most of the year either alone or in groups of up to twelve.

9.1 Association and Social behaviour

Yaks are gregarious in nature. They like to stay in herds. Herd size varies from 20 to 200, including female yak and calves. Old male yak are solitary and sometimes live in herds of five. It is highly unusual to lose an animal from attack by wild animals, as the yak protect each other. When grazing, they are never far apart from each other.

As calving occurs during the summer months, thus in early spring, herds increase in size and are found around grassy grounds, where they are attracted by newly sprouting grasses. Herds of yaks are led by a lead yak. Herders communicate with the yaks by making clicking sounds with their tongues.

Yaks are extremely observant and aware of their surroundings, and are suspicious of strangers. They are not aggressive, but rather are quite easy to move and direct with the help of a long stick as a visual aid and guide. Yak will even find their way back to the campsite without a herder - if it is not too far away.

Yaks are a herd animal and form social groups. The males join with the herd at breeding season otherwise remain alone. They like to roam as they graze. They also prefer grazing and roam in the middle of the night. They can be flighty when one senses danger and for no apparent reason, the whole herd may storm off because one does. This is perhaps one of the more dangerous aspects of yak herding. They are big, strong and instinctual when startled.

9.2 Reactive behaviour

Yak are usually and fairly docile but its not always true. Various reports are found regarding attack of the yak. If any person tries to interrupt their personal space, they warn by grunting and head shaking before taking more aggressive measures. Yak are easily frightened and vigilant to attack by wild animals, wolves in particular. The yak will form a defensive position and fight off aggressors. They panic easily. If one yak panics often the whole herd follows suit. Herders sometimes purposely panic the lead yak, so that herd acts as a snowplow and clears the way.

Owing to the highly reactive nervous system, yak easily gets excited and quickly reacts to changes in the environment. The sexual activity of female yak is suppressed by heat, lower altitudes (or a higher oxygen content in the ambient air), low-growing grasses in the pasture and other unfavourable conditions. They are so sensitive that the presence of a herdsman in the vicinity of the animals interferes not only with the reflexes of the animals but also with their grazing. Yaks try to keep out of sight of man; their sexual reflexes are suppressed in man's presence. Therefore, in the breeding season prolonged driving and other factors which may bother them should be avoided.

9.3 Sexual behaviour

Males and females of differ conspicuously in their size, appearance and mating behaviour.

9.3.1 Male

Bulls usually stay alone except the breeding season. During the mating season, the bulls join the herd and fight other bulls for mating with the females. Mating season begins in September. Bulls can pick up the scent of females on heat at a distance of several kilometres - even 10 km have been reported by the farmers. They claims that a male yak can detect its female counterpart in estrus in a block of a district.

Some males stay with female herds throughout the year (Schaller 1998), but others live alone or in bachelor groups until rut in summer—as late as July for domestic yaks (Wiener *et al.*, 2003). At some point, older males may become less competitive in obtaining mates than prime males and may live alone or in small groups apart from other groups (Harris, 2008). During rut, males do not establish a territory or *harem* apart from a herd or each other, but rather they 'wander day and night' and attempt to tend and breed receptive females within existing herds (Wiener *et al.*, 2003).

Yak are seasonal breeder. As rut commences, males maintain a dominance hierarchy by fighting each other and attain maximum breeding performance at 5–10 years, at least among domestic breeds (Wiener and Long, 2003). Aggressive behavior among males in rut is intense. Considerable scarring, wounds, and horn damage on male wild yaks found during rut-induced fights. Indirect threats involve lateral displays that emphasize the shoulder hump and mantle of hair by standing head to head or head to tail 3–6 m apart for about 5 min; direct threats include charges with lowered heads and head-to-head sparring that can last 15 min (Schaller, 1998). Rutting male wild yaks frequently wallow or rolling on dry ground, sometimes while defecating and urinating, which distinguishes them from other *Bos* but parallels behavior of Bison. Other rutting behaviors include grunting, bellowing, horning the ground and vegetation, rubbing the face and neck on the ground, and teeth grinding (Schaller, 1998). Copulation is abrupt and of short duration.

Courtship behaviour

When female is in heat, several males fight each other to obtain the custody of the female. Strongest bull gets the dominant position in this event. Usually oldest but virile bull gets the strongest position. However, other strongest yet younger bulls also get the opportunity for mating in a very few occasion. Very young bulls not at all win the competition for mating until they are four years old. After that they seldom get the opportunity provided they have some fighting experience in the previous year. As the strongest bull become older, the bull become feeble and fails to retain the mating position in the hierarchy of the herd. The bulls do not try to mate and leave the herd. After the age of eight years, yak bulls start to lose to younger bulls in the competition for females. Older bulls are replaced by another younger and stronger bull, and which is usually before the daughter of older bull reaches at breeding age. This competitive event may also help in reducing the chance of inbreeding in the herd. When the breeding season is over, bulls spend winter and spring alone.

The fighting process during mating is the one aspect of natural selection. It provides strength to the coming generation for the survival in a harsh and often unfriendly environment.

Mating behaviour

Yak bulls are sexually very active. After establishment of dominant position in the herd, bull mate with the female several times a day. The mating process is so focused that bull will not attack other companion, unless strongly provoked. As the process of mating continues the dominant/strongest bull engage in mating frequently. They hardly graze or take any feed during this time. Day by day their body condition deteriorates as a result of their sexual activity ceases over the mating season. As a result of that less dominant males get the opportunity for mating.

9.3.2 Female

Most yak start their oestrus in the early morning or in the evening and only rarely at other times of day. Detection of oestrus by the herdsman is a very difficult task. Changes in the appearance of the reproductive organs are more obvious than behavioural changes, although these also occur. The vulva becomes swollen and the vagina reddens. Mucus is discharged from the vulva in a majority of females in oestrous, but in some animals it may not be observed. Other signs like dilatation of vagina and cervix, raising her tail, frequent urination etc. Estrus females stop eating, become excited, and occasionally attempt to mount other females (Sarkar and Prakash, 2005). Like cattle, at the time of oestrous in lactating yak daily milk yield decline. Sometimes farmer prefer a particular yak bull to be used for mating and mass mating is not practiced. Then detection of heat is requires with the use of a teaser bull. Katzina and Maturova (1989) observed that signs of heat in yak are less obvious than in other cattle, and detection by herdsmen is unreliable.

9.4 Parturient behaviour

Maternal behviour plays an important role in the social organization and preservation of a particular species. For the offspring, behaviour of the mother is critical, not only for life itself but also for the adjustment to the environment into which it is born. Mother is the chief source of learning. By her response to the separate acts of the young, the mother can be said to shape its behavioural patterns.

As the time of parturition approaches, the female yak behaves unusually. They withdraw themselves from the herd. They seek sheltered spots such as a depression in the ground or a ditch at a distance from the herd. Typical behaviour of the yak during labour includes lying on her side and standing up again for delivery when a pure yak calf is carried. When a hybrid calf is carried, the female will deliver the calf while lying on her side - presumably on account of the larger size of the calf and the longer time needed for the delivery (Cai Li, 1989). Most of the cases parturition takes place during day time. It may be postulated that the pattern is the most suitable for the survival of the new born; because predators can be easily seen in the broad day light and new born can establish a close bond with mother.

Parturition takes place as effortless, problem free, and finished within very short time. Parturition process completes within 40 minutes. Naval cord is broken automatically when its mother stands up after delivery or by the yak calf falling down. The placenta is ejected usually within half an hour. However, in some cases it may extent upto six hours after parturition.

Dam stands up very shortly after delivery. They start licking the newborn usually starting from the head. Licking cleans the birth fluids from the young and possible marks them for recognition. Dam licks the newborn calf for about ten minutes. During grooming, both dam and offspring vocalize and this is important in the development of the parent-offspring bond. Only a short period (called critical period) of contact is needed to establish a bond which enables the mother to identify its own offspring from the others. It appears that in this initial period the dam that has given birth approaches any young animals and will become attach to it. The attachment is learned. Few hours during this period, maternal behaviour is under hormonal control but after that new born calf has to provide cues that stimulate the dam to remain maternal. During this period, dam dislike her offspring to be approached by any stranger and the vicinity is closely observed by her and reacts instantly to save the young.

9.5 Neonatal behaviour

Just after birth of the calf, dam licks the newborn calf, after which the calf attempts to stand up. The behaviour of the dam is coordinated with the movement of new born calf, which is trying to stand up before it can orientate and even reach the mammary gland. As the new born calf begins to stand, it moves forward and it is attracted towards any object. As dam is the nearest object, the calf moves down the flank of the dam and puts its head under the abdomen. When the head of the calf touches the abdomen of its dam, there is a reflex movement which brings neonate's head up and the nose makes contact with the body of the dam. The calf assumes a crouched stance, with legs spread and shoulder lowered, which allows it to bunt upwards at the udder. It appears to nose and lick the ventral surface of dam, with its steps forwards, it gradually progresses towards the udder. The udder bunting functions in the stimulation of milk let-down. The calf sucks their dam just after 20-30 minutes of birth. The calf starts running in minutes. They sleep a lot in the first day. The event of parturition exposes the newborn animals to a greater variety of stimuli than it has encountered before. Therefore, the neonate has to learn many aspects of the environment very quickly. Investigation is the major part of the young calf's behaviour.

First week of the calf's life are packed with rapid learning. Presence of the dam and their maternal care seems to provide a sense of security so that calf moves close to their dam when alarmed. New born calves at their early days show capricious behaviour as spontaneous act of play. Infant play appears to be most important for the development of early social organization. Solitary play can take the form of running around in confined area, a form of exercise. It also acts as a means of practicing and perfecting adult behavioural skills necessary for defense and certain patterns of movement. Play is valuable tool for the development of normal behaviour. Only healthy calves are engaged in playing and its absence may be an indicator of improper health. Dam's behaviour influences the calf's behaviour from an early age, particularly in searching for food and in alarm responses to possible danger. The survival of the calf solely depends upon its mother, which provides nourishment, grooming, protection and guidance for survival in this harsh environmental condition.

Weaning is well accepted and practiced by the farmers. At the time of weaning they only produce simple grunts, no bellowing or mooing. Either dam or calf does not show any type of stress due to weaning. If the farmer raises hybrids they weaned the offspring early to harvest more and more milk but in case of pure yak, its not done strictly as pure yak hardly reared for milk production. Offspring from pure yak, rather not weaned just to make it healthier and assumed to be slaughtered next year which will yield higher meat.

9.6 Ingestive behaviour

Yak has a square tongue, broad muzzle and mobile lips that allow them to graze close to the ground, where other domestic animal can not graze. Yak are browsers and grazers; they thrive on brush and marginal pasture. They are extremely efficient eaters and simply browse on whatever is available. They are better than other animals at digging below icy snow to get grass. Some yaks spend so much time grazing on their own they become semi-wild, although they are domesticated.

Grazing habit

Although grazing method is different in cattle and sheep, one peculiarity of the yak is that they can graze like cattle as well as sheep. Like cattle yak can graze long grasses, using their tongue and like sheep they can also graze short grass and creeping stems, and roots of grass using their incisor teeth and lips. Yak can also take tender branches of shrubs in alpine bush meadow. Normally yak has the ability to avoid poisonous or thorny plants as recorded instances of poisoning are very rare. However, there are reports of extensive pyrrolizidine alkaloid poisoning in a part of Bhutan. This plant was almost certainly eaten by the yak because of overstocking of the pastures concerned, leading to overgrazing (Winter *et al.*, 1992). When the ground is covered with snow, as it typically is for long periods, yak will paw through quite thick snow layers, using both head and face to help them to gain access to the wilted vegetation underneath.

In the spring, yak will graze green shoots not more than 2-3 cm above the ground - though it would be surprising if they could not graze more closely than that if necessary. In addition, the yak take stems and leaves from the residual wilted grass still available in the spring. The yak graze mostly in the morning and evening. Due to the sparseness of vegetation in its environment, the yak must travel long distances to obtain its needed nourishment.

Rumination

Like other ruminant yak also ruminate. They follow four periods of rumination in each day when they graze in the day only. They start grazing in the early morning. First rumination initiates two hours after the start of morning grazing. Second period of rumination is around noon, when the ambient temperature is high and yak stop grazing. Third period of rumination takes place about two hours before the animals are driven from the pasture back to the campsite. Fourth period of rumination is in the evening. Rumination periods generally last between 0.8 and 1.9 hours. If yak are allowed to graze throughout the day and night, the periods of rumination are different. In case of pack yak, the periods of rumination fit in with the timing and intensity of the work being performed. Yak seldom ruminate at night, when they lie in a state of light sleep. In other types of cattle, the frequency of contractions when the animal is resting or ruminating may be only half the rate during feeding.

Intake time

The grazing time of yak is affected by season, weather, type and quality of grazing and the structure of the herd in terms of age and sex (Zhang Hongwu, *et al.*, 1985). The intake time varies between 34 percent and 80 percent of the total time available for grazing. The rest of the time they are engaged in walking, resting and drinking. Normally, lactating yak herds spend more time grazing than do mixed herds. However, in herds of mixed age, where females have young calves at foot, the grazing rhythm is disturbed as the calves suckle and also learn to graze. Under such conditions, the intake time may be curtailed.

Bite rate

Unlike other pasture animals yak shows relatively little variation in the bite rate. It varies between 0.8 to 1.1 mouthfuls per second. However, intake varies with season, sward height and other factors. Intake ranges from around 28 kg to 38 kg herbage over a period of ten hours in the summer to only 13 kg or less in the same period when grazing wilted grass in the cold season in adults. The energy and protein intakes are adequate to meet maintenance, work and production, but in the later parts of the winter and the early spring they fall below the requirements. Yak then lose weight and condition and this is true for the offsprings. Milk to the offspring as well as fodder/ feed availability to the dam declines at the end of winter resulting in decreased milk production and severe climatic conditions force the young one to thrive on low body weight, body condition with poor feed otherwise death may follow.

9.7 Investigative/Exploratory behaviour

Yaks are very sure-footed—even on narrow, step, rock-strewn trails with heavy loads on their back. They walk confidently through raging streams and along mountain paths with thousand-meter drops. However, they are notoriously slow and stubborn. They do not prefer to walk on broken ground, rocky places and glaciers, but are good swimmers. A newly-born calf can easily cross icy mountain streams by attaching firmly onto the tail of elder yak. Due to the sparseness of vegetation in the very high altitude, alpine and sub-alpine region, yak must travel long distances to obtain its needed nourishment.

As the summer season starts, yak engage in grazing in the summer pasture. With the advancement of the warm season, they move into the upper reaches until autumn. Throughout the summer they remain there. They return back to lower elevations in the valleys and water logged areas and wander for grasses in wastelands during winter.

Depending upon the pasture condition and season the speed with which yak moves varies. On the start of the day they are usually faster than later part of the day. They are slow in the pasture where vegetation is of good quality. In the warm season they are slow in the pasture in comparison the cold season. In the adverse climatic condition like snow or hail storms, yak can be seen to run over the pasture, in bursts of speed up to 57 m per minute which is to four times the normal speed at the start of the day. They generally move 3–5 km/day while grazing and rest under cliffs.

If the road was doubtful, yak raisers drive a yak up it before them. As yak is sure footed animals, they would detect any ravines and crevasses. When the road is covered by thick snow and it is unfit for the movement of the men and horses, then yak herd drive ahead of the group. Yak trampled the drifts down and made them a regular highway. That's why they are called "biological snow plough".

9.8 Epimeletic (care giving) behaviour

Yak has strong maternal instinct. The dam generally licks the newborn calf for about ten minutes. Soon after, the calf attempts to stand up and suck. Again, differences in behaviour have been observed between dams delivering pure-bred yak and F1 calves. They show that time intervals are markedly longer when a F1 calf is involved than when pure yak calves are born. The survival of the calf is purely depending upon the care provided by the mother. Shortly after birth, the dam is intensely protective of her calf and may attack person coming close. Bonding of dam and calf depends mainly on smelling and licking. Longer times of parturition and dystokia militate against such bonding. Yak cows can distinguish their calves by smell from among quite large groups of calves. In the calfhood, the calf solely depends on their mother's milk. The dam provides milk to their calves at the cost of decreasing body condition or losing body weight especially during winter and spring season. Yak calf remains with the mother for about a year.

9.9 Resting behaviour

Usually animals take rest when time not used for other activities. At their calfhood, young yak gets very little time for suckling. They spend greater proportion of time of the day and night for rest. As the yak calf grows, they start taking solid feeds and subsequently the rest period starts declining. As yaks are maintained in free range system, they spend most of the time for waking for the search of feed materials. In summer, they usually graze in the morning and evening, while they take rest in and around noon.

Yaks generally sleep standing up. Yak takes rest when they stands. This would minimize heat loss from lying on the cold wet ground. They love the snow and sometime they sleep on it.

References

Cai Li 1989. Sichuan Yak. Chengdu, Sichuan Publication House.

Frazer, A.F. 1985. Ethology of farm animals. Elsevier Science Publishing Company. New York.

Harris, R.B. 2008. Wildlife conservation in China: preserving the habitat of China's Wild West. M. E. Sharpe, Armonk, New York.

Katzina, E.V. and Maturova, E.T. 1989. The reproductive function of yak cows. Doklady vsesoyuznoi ordena lenina akademii sel'skokhozyaistvennykh naukim V.I. Lenina, 4: 26-29. (Cited from CAB Animal Breeding Abstracts, 58: 352.)

Sarkar, M. and B. S. Prakash. 2005. Timing of ovulation in relation to onset of estrus and LH peak in yak (*Poephagus grunniens L.*). Animal Reproduction Science 86:353–362.

Schaller, G. B. 1998. Wildlife of the Tibetan steppe. University of Chicago Press, Chicago, Illinois.

Wiener, G., J. Han, and R. Long (Eds.). 2003. The yak. 2nd ed. Regional Office for Asia and the Pacific, Food and Agriculture Organization, Bangkok, Thailand.

Winter, H., A.A. Seawright, J. Hrdlicka, U. Tshewang and B.J. Gurung. 1992. Pyrrolizidine alkaloid poisoning of yaks *(Bos grunniens)* and confirmation by recovery of pylloric metabolites from formalin-fixed liver tissue. Research in Veterinary Science, 52, 187-194.

Zhang Hongwu, Zhao Yibin and Lei Huangzhang 1985. Studies on ecological reaction of yak and its hybrid during pasturing in cold season. Journal of China yak, (3), 15-21.

□□□

Chapter 10

Diseases of Yak

In the ancient times, attempts to control diseases were associated with Apollo in Greece. The Apollo was regarded as the God of healing in Greece. Asclepios, the son of Apollo, founded temples where sick peoples were treated through prayer, message etc. The Greek physicians had the opinion that human body is maintained through equilibrium of 'humours' i.e., yellow bile, black bile, phlegm and blood. Later, the Father of Medicine, Hippocrates gave emphasis the theory that if there is an imbalance of the body 'humours' there will be disease. Lastly in the nineteenth century there was a tremendous development of physiology, morphology and the science of deviation from physiology or pathology. In brief, any deviation from normal physiology or physiological condition will be considered as disease. It indicates the inability to perform the normal physiological functions through nutrition and other environmental condition are maintained at optimum level.

Broadly the disease may be classified as specific and non- specific disease based on etiology of the disease. Specific disease, where it has got a definite identity and are produced by a particular pathogen or factor whereas the non- specific diseases are caused by a number of pathogen and / or factors. Specific disease may be sub- divided into contagious (spread by intimate contact) and infectious (caused by living infecting organism). However, all contagious diseases are infectious but all infectious diseases may not be contagious in nature.

The other class of disease may be deficiency and metabolic disease which are caused by deficiency of any nutrient or imbalance of internal products inside the body. For readers point of view, we will discuss the disease encounters by yak as viral, bacterial, endoparasitic and metabolic diseases.

10.1 Viral diseases

Foot and Mouth disease (FMD)

FMD or apthous fever is an acute febrile and highly contagious disease in cattle, buffalo and yak (with other cloven footed animals). It is characterized by vesicular eruptions in and around mouth, feet, udder and teat. The disease causes high morbidity resulting in heavy economic loss in cattle and buffalo. It is caused picorna virus (RNA virus) group and several strains have identified viz., 'O', 'A' , 'C', SAT 1, SAT 2, SAT 3 and Asia1.

The disease is not fatal but morbidity is 100 percent and the symptoms are high rise of temperature, generalized malaise, depression, apathy to feed and water. Vesicles appear after febrile condition in buccal cavity, soft palate, tongue, udder and teat and leg. On rupture of the vesicles, ulcers appear and profuse salivation found in the affected animals. There may be abortion of pregnant animal and mastitis in lactating animals. Subsequently, animal recovers but show certain abnormalities like panting, anaemia, overgrowth of hair etc which are called as sequel of FMD. Prasad (1978) reported an outbreak of this disease in Himachal yak and strain O was isolated from the infected animals.

Treatment

There is no specific treatment except the symptomatic one. Antiseptic mouth wash with potassium permanganate ($KMnO_4$), boric acid and glycerine may be done to prevent secondary bacterial infection. Control can only effectively done by vaccination of animals regularly to the livestock in a particular area. Joshi *et al.* (1997) reported a number of outbreaks in different parts of Nepal among yak and hybrids of yak with local cattle. They state that quarantine of affected animals is used in alpine regions of Nepal with the intention of allowing the lesions to heal and that vaccination, though effective, is not widely used.

10.1.1 Infectious Bovine Rhinotracheitis (IBR)

The Infectious Bovine Rhinotracheitis is caused by a herpes virus I or bovine herpes virus and characterized by high rise of temperature, rhinitis, dyspnoea, kerato- conjunctivitis and can cause abortion in severe cases. The virus multiplies in the upper respiratory tract and causes inflammatory changes like rhinitis, laryngitis and tracheitis. In some cases, this may cause pneumonia and conjunctivitis. The virus may enter brain tissues fromnasal mucosa via trigemianal nerves and produce meningo- encephalitis. The virus may also produce changes in placenta and cause abortion. Rahman *et al.* (2007a) observed infectious bovine rhinotracheitis in yaks revealed that the overall prevalence of IBR in yaks was 40.80 percent. The prevalence was higher among females (42.05percent) than male yaks (37.84percent). The prevalence of IBR was highest in yak cows (54.39 percent) followed by yak bulls (37.84 percent) and yak heifers (28.57 percent). The prevalence of IBR was higher (43.53 percent) among animals reared at a lower altitude (West Kameng district, 2751 masl) than those (35.00 percent) reared at higher altitude (Tawang district, 3500 masl).

Treatment

There is no specific treatment for the disease but to control the secondary bacterial infection, broad spectrum antibiotic and to maintain electrolyte balance fluid therapy should be done. Quarantine of affected animal and vaccination of animals may be done to control the outbreak of the disease.

10.1.2 Rinderpest

Yak are highly susceptible to Rinderpest or cattle plague with reported mortality rates of 90 - 100 percent. In India, the disease has been eradicated through vaccination. The disease is characterized by necrotic stomatitis, gastro-enteritis, dehydration and destruction of lymphocytes. The disease is caused by RNA virus belonging to the paramixo group. As the virus has got special affinity to lymphoid tissues, epithelial cells of GI tract and respiratory tract, the symptoms accordingly appeared in the respective organs. The disease may be seen in 4 stages i.e., incubation stage, prodormal stage, mucosal stage (most symptoms are seen in this stage) and finally the convalescent stage where mostly animal recovers from the infection.

Treatment

There is no effective treatment against the disease but rinderpest antisera may be administered to save valuable animal. Antibiotics and fluid therapy may be adopted to prevent the fluid loss of the animal and bacterial infection.

10.1.3 Viral diarrhoea/mucosal disease

Bovine viral diarrhea is an acute, sub acute or inapparent contagious disease characterized by high rise of temperature and severe diarrhea. This is caused by RNA virus belongs to toga virus and susceptible hosts are cattle, deer, buffalo and wild ruminants. Direct and indirect contact with infected animals spread the disease to other animal/ herd. Contaminated feed and water may act as source of contamination, through infected trough or other appliances may spread the disease. The acute form is serious in nature and characterized by high rise of temperature and it may be bi- phasic in nature. There may be anorexia, depression, tachycardia and polydipsia along with nasal discharge. Animal may die due to septicemia and severe dehydration. Mild for is characterized by fever, for short duration, loss milk yield, transient diarrhea and infrequent mouth lesion.

Treatment

There is no fruitful treatment against the viral infection but to safeguard the animal supportive therapy is essential, fluid therapy, antibiotic and chemotherapeutics are helpful to combat secondary bacterial infection. To prevent the further spreading of the virus strict hygienic and sanitary measures to be adopted in the farm.

Other viral diseases found in yak which are not economically important under Indian point of view. Though there is no organized study under Indian situation as far as viral diseases are concerned.

10.2 Bacterial diseases

10.2.1 Anthrax

This is a zoonotic disease and also known as wool sorter's disease, splenic fever, charbon and tarka, characterized by high rise of temperature, depression, distressed breathing and death in extreme condition. Following death there is oozing of blood from natural orifices. Carcass decomposes rapidly with formation of gas and distension of abdomen. Rigor mortis absent from carcass and blood is dark red or black in appearance and does not clot rapidly. The disease caused by bacteria *Bacillus anthracis*, which produces 3 types of extra cellular toxin viz., factor I (edema toxin), II (protecting antigen) and III (lethal factor). When the bacteria is exposed to air, forms spore which is resistant to cold, hot, drying and any chemical treatment and it is remain viable for many years in soil. The pH and humidity of the soil have got some clinical bearance on spread of the disease. It has been pointed out that alkaline soil is a factor for soil borne outbreaks. Animals while graze in the infected pasture pick up the infection through ingestion or through breach in the oral mucosa or skin.

Treatment

In per acute case, no scope of treatment but in other cases may be done with penicillin or other broad spectrum antibiotic as these drugs are effective against the bacteria. Vaccination is the best procedure to control the outbreak but the adjacent areas of the dead and infected animals should be thoroughly disinfected by applying 3 percent acetic acid, 10 percent KOH or formaline. The dead animals along with hides, skin, wool, bone meal etc should be buried properly as the spore become viable for longer period and infect the handling men/ women causing cutaneous abscess.

10.2.2 Brucellosis

This infectious disease, also known as Bang's disease, undulant fever, malta fever and Mediterranean fever which has importance throughout the world, is common among yak and its hybrids. Concern with Brucellosis is made the greater by the fact that it is readily transmitted to humans.

The disease is caused by *Brucella abortus, B. melitensis* are aerobic but require added CO_2 for growth in growth medium and transmitted through ingestion of contaminated with discharges of aborted foetus/ fetal membrane and food and water. The infection may also transmitted through flies, ticks, rat, dog and infected bulls. *B. abortus* has got special affinity to invade gravid uterus, mammary gland, testes, lymph node and joints. The organism gain access through mucous membrane of the oropharynx, upper respiratory tract, conjunctival mucosa, abraded skin, cervix etc. Rahman et al. (2007b) observed seroprevalence of brucellosis in yaks (*Poephagus grunniens*) and revealed that the overall prevalence of brucellosis in yaks was 16.0 percent in Arunachal Pradesh, India. The prevalence was higher among females (18.18 percent) compared to male yaks (12.81 percent). The prevalence of brucellosis was highest in yak cows (22.81 percent) followed by yak bulls (12.81 percnet) and yak heifers (12.29 percent). The prevalence of brucellosis was higher (18.82percent) among animals reared at a lower altitude (West Kameng district, 2751 masl) than those (10.00percent) reared at higher altitude (Tawang district, 3500 masl).

10.2.3 Colibacillosis

Commonly known as calf scours caused by *Eschericia coli* in new born calves. In some herds, 30 - 40 percent of calves, particularly the spring-born, develop profuse diarrhoea though this does not necessarily impair the general condition of the animals. The stools are of a thin, pasty to watery consistency, sometimes containing blood. Traditionally, affected animals are given a drink made from medicinal herbs. However, scours in young calves, mostly from birth to few days of age. A report by Lensch (1996) indicates that a mortality rate due to *Eschericia coli* infection in yak calves was 20 - 30 percent.

Treatment

In general, recovery rates are high if anti-bacterial treatment is given, but such treatment is not widespread. Assessing the degree of dehydration, fluid therapy should be initiated. Oral rehydration solution used for human being may be adopted. To control such condition, colostrum should be fed within 24 hrs of birth and strict hygienic condition in and around the shed should be maintained.

10.2.4 Leptospirosis

It is a zoonotic disease, which causes a generalized but serious illness in yak, characterized by high rise of temperature, haemoglobinuria, icterus and abortion. The etiological agent is *Leptospira* sp. There are around 200 serologically distinct Leptospira. Transmission of the organism takes place through direct contact with the infected urine or ingestion of urine contaminated water or food. The organism enters through abraded skin and mucous membrane in to the blood and various visceral organs. If the animals can overcome the initial attack, the organism settles into liver and cause hepatic dysfunction. Lesions in kidneys are also common in most of the cases which may lead to ureamic coma and death.

Treatment

Drug of choice in case of leptospirosis is penicillin, streptomycin or tetracycline. Supportive therapy is to be followed for normal kidney and liver function. All possible measures should be taken to avoid contamination by excreta of infected and wild animals. During high hill grazing animals may bring the infection to herd, in that case ailing animals must be segregated from rest of the herd. The animal should be diagnosed for cause of disease and accordingly treatment to be done.

10.2.5 Mastitis

Mastitis occurs in yak, but it is believed that the incidence is less than among dairy cattle, perhaps on account of the relatively low milk yield of yak and the suckling of calves. Joshi *et al.* (1997) reported that in a study of mastitis in yak herds in Nepal, the bacteria isolated from the milk were mainly *Staphylococcus aureus, Streptococcus agalactiae* and other *Streptococcus spp.* and *E. coli.*

10.2.6 Haemorrhagic septisemia

This disease is prevalent in yak-producing areas and caused by *Pasteurella multocida,* a gram negative bacteria, characterized by high rise of temperature, depression, pneumonia, pleuritis and found to occur after stress such as transportation from one place to another. The disease is transported through contact with infected animals, inhalation of contaminated droplets. Joshi (1982) noted the occurrence of haemorrhagic septicaemia among hybrids of yak with local cattle in many districts of Nepal but made the point that these were in the lower and middle hill regions where the disease can be virulent and result in high mortality and that the incidence was much more limited in the higher alpine areas. Pal (1993) also quoted the occurrence of the disease among yak in Arunachal Pradesh, India.

Treatment

High dose of penicillin may be the drug of choice but for effective control vaccination is essential.

10.2.7 Salmonellosis

The disease is common among yak in China, mostly young calves are the victim of the bacteria (*S. typhimurium, S. dublin* and *S. newport* have been isolated). Hygienic and clean environment at the site of shed may be one of the best control measure. Other than this, sulphur drugs may be administered to combat the disease.

10.2.8 Tuberculosis

Yak are susceptible to the bovine strain of *Mycobacterium tuberculosis*. Although the disease is known to occur in yak, there is little quantified information available and no control schemes are in place. In Tibet around 12.7 percent of animals are suffering from the disease, but some of these showed no visible lesions. In India, mass examination have been done to quantify the number of affected animals but certainly observing the infection among human beings, some animals may suffer from the disease.

10.2.9 Contagious bovine pleuropneumonia

This disease is caused by *Mycoplasma mycoides* and occurs among yak, between two and ten years old, principally in winter and spring when the animals are more closely confined than in the summer. Though vaccination is an effective option for control, it is not widely practiced.

10.3 Parasitic diseases

Ectoparasites

Ticks, fleas, lice and mites

These have all been found in yak, though herdsmen do not, in general, recognize their importance or the irritant effect on the animals.

Ticks: A report by Biswas *et al.* (1994) documents infestations with ticks of five genera, among yak is tracts of Arunachal Pradesh of India and lists the types found and the sites os infection on the animal. Tick infestation is at its height in the rainy season from May to September. Ecological planning is recommended for tick control and should take into account seasonal variations, range of hosts, and known infected areas. The traditional method used by Mongolians of moving the cattle and yak to more or less tick-free grazing land during the summer months, largely protects the animals from (heavy) tick infestation. Joshi

(1982) also referred to ticks among yak in Nepal and draws attention to the possible disease transmission caused by them there.

Lice: The report of Biswas *et al.* (1994) also provides evidence of infestation by lice of one genus in Arunashal Pradesh. There are apparently on report of this parasite in yak from elsewhere.

Mites: of a number of different families have been recorded in yak and yak hybrids in Nepal (Joshi, 1982). The main families are *Psoroptidae* and *Sarcoptidae* and cause the disease commonly called "mange". The clinical symptoms are persistent itching and chronic inflammation of large areas of the skin, especially of the back. Like in Nepal, Yu also observed mite infestations of yak in China (mainly yak calves of one to two years old).

10.3.1 Endoparasites

All India Network Programme on Gastrointestinal parasitism in yak in Sikkim (Rahman *et al.*, 2009) reported that around 21 percent animals were positive for several internal parasites. The most common parasite was strongyle (17 percent) followed by *Eimeria* sp (4.5 percent), Strongyloides (4.4 percent), Moniezia (3 percent), Trichuris (2.9 percent), Amphistome (0.5 percent) and Dicrocoelium sp (0.3 percent). The occurrence of gastrointestinal parasitism was found to be higher (30 percent) among yak population reared at a lower altitude with low humidity than those reared at higher altitude with high humidity (19 percent). There are some common endoparasites discussed below.

Fasciolasis

This is a common parasite in yak China, Nepal but occurance of the parasite under Indian subcontinent is very few. This is caused by Fasciola hepatica and causes huge economic loss to the farmers.

Babesiasis (tick-borne)

This disease is caused by *Babesia bigemina* a protozoan parasite. In Aba prefecture of Sichuan province in 1981, 549 cases of yak infected with the disease were found and 273 of them died. In 1985, the disease broke out elsewhere in Sichuan province where around 500 yak died from it (Yu *et al.*, 1989). The organism is transmitted by ticks, and the symptoms are fever and haemoglobinuria.

Roundworms

A report by Liu (1994), from studies in Tibet, suggested that roundworm infestations and the associated larvae may be a common problem in yak, though not as extensive as among the sheep on the same pastures. Many genera of roundworm were isolated (Liu, 1994), but the prevalence of different genera varied with the time of year. He noted that routine antiparasitic treatments were restricted to government yak farms and a few selected private farms but that the majority of yak were not involved in any treatment programme because worm infestation does not cause visible symptoms that might alert yak herders to a problem. Wangdi (1996) examined faecal samples collected at random from 26 adult yak and 81 yak calves from western Bhutan. The results showed that in the adult yak, 19 percent were positive for *Strongyle spp.*, while among the calves 37 percent were positive for *Strongyle spp.*, 2 percent for *Coccidia spp.* and also 2 percent for *Trichuris spp.* Pal (1993) quoted one study on yak in Sikkim showing 62 percent of yak infected with helminths. Another report based on a study conducted by the National Research Centre on yak in India in 1995 indicated that of the 63 yak faecal samples examined in Arunachal Pradesh, 32 were positive for various helminth eggs (*Trichuris, Strongyles,* hookworms, *Dicrocoelium* and *Ascaris*).

10.4 Metabolic and deficiency diseases

10.4.1 Bloat

The condition is also known as tympany or hoven and results in either due to excessive production of gas or physical obstruction in the process of eructation gas from rumen. It is a clinical condition where rumen and reticulum are filled with gasses of fermentation due to excessive highly fermentable feeds, fodders like lucerne, berseem, clover

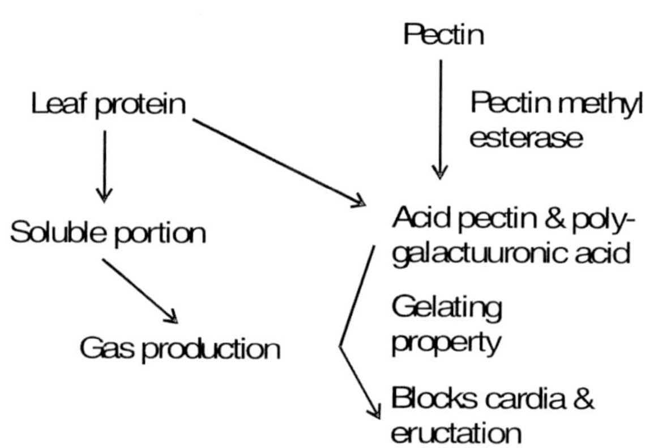

etc, some time gas bubbles remains intimately adhered with the ingesta, the condition called frothy bloat. Mechanism of occurance of bloat is shown below

Symptoms of generalized enlargement of rumen (left side of the animal), extension head, protrusion of tongue, restlessness, anorexia, ruminal motolity goes high initially followed by hypo- motility and later atony may be observed. If the animals not treated in time, animal may die.

Treatment

Trocarization to remove the gas, carminative mixtures and mineral or vegetable oil for immediate treatment. Dimethicone suspension (bloatosil, bloatonil) may also be the drug of choice for bloat.

10.4.2 Acidosis

Accidental ingestion of escessive carbohydrate containing grains like rice, wheat, barley potato etc there is formation of lactic acid in huge quantities in rumen, resulting in lowering pH from 6.8 to about 5.0 or so. This results in accumulation of more fluid form rumen wall and circulatory system due to high osmolarity of lactate. This may lead to dehydration, oligourea and anurea causing ruminal stasis and laminitis.

Treatment

1. Sodium bicarbonate 2.5-5.0 percent solution 500 ml to 1 lt through i/v route, 7 percent solution 200-500 ml.
2. pH correction by $MgCO_3$, MgO, $Mg(OH)_2$ or $NaHCO_3$
3. Corticosteroid to prevent shock.

10.4.3 Ketosis

It is a condition of relative or absolute lack of carbohydrate in the hepatic cells leading to β oxidation of fats, resulting in production of ketone bodies i.e., acetoacetic acid, β hydroxyl butyrate and acetone. All carbohydrate feeds in the rumen on fermentation produces VFAs i.e, acetate, propionate an butyrate along with some branched chain fatty acids. Among which, acetate and butyrate are ketogenic whereas propionate are the major one and produced in the ratio of 75:25. The ratio if changed due to feeding or any other reason caused ketosis.

It may be primary where starvation/ underfed for longer period and secondary where any disease or syndrome causes starvation to the animal. But clinically ketosis may be of four type i.e., alimentary, spontaneous, nervous and milk fever type.

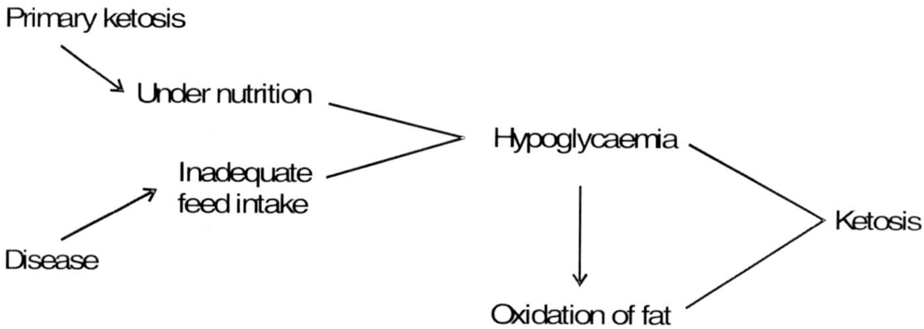

Treatment

1. 500- 800 ml of 40-50 percent dextrose solution through i/v route.
2. Glycerine of glycerol @100 gm twice daily for 2-3 days.
3. Sodium propionate@ 100-200 g once daily for 3 days.

10.4.4 Milk fever

It is also known as parturient peresis, is a metabolic disease occurring mostly within 72 hrs of parturition in adult female and is characterized by hypocalcaemia, changes in neuromuscular tone ranging from fine tremor in early stages to peresis, recumbancy, circulatory collapse and ultimately diminution of conciseness. Temperature is generally subnormal in advance stages. There is muscle weakness and flaccidity of muscles. There is found in the eye and muzzle. Hypocalcaemia may be termed as deficiency disease but since the deficiency of Ca in feed is not the main factor of disease and there are other causal factors, the disease termed as metabolic disease rather than a deficiency disease. In case of low intake of Ca and excretion through milk in high producing animals leads to the disease.

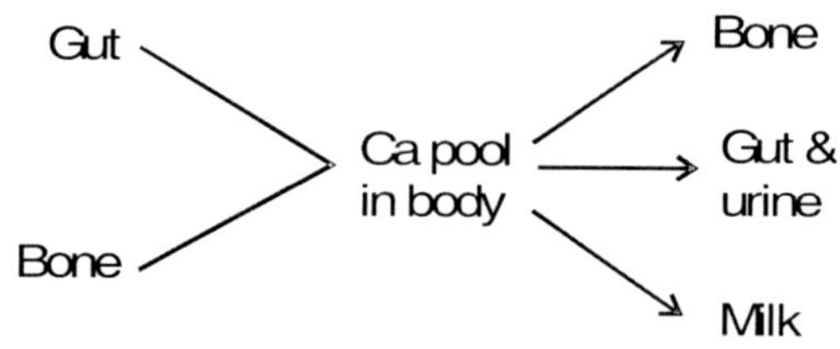

Treatment

Effort should be to supplement Ca to the infected animals. If its done in proper stage, lateral incumbency for longer time may cause death of the animal.

1. Ca borogluconate through i/v route @ 250-500 ml
2. Ca Mg borogluconate same dose.
3. Vitamin D3 or cholecalcipherol single dose i/m route @ 8mg prior to 3 - 4 days calving in high producing animals.

10.4.5 Grass tetany

Metabolic disease of cattle, sheep, goat and even horse characterized by hyper- aesthesia, in coordination and convulsion as a result of altered Mg homeostasis. Young green pasture is generally poor in Mg deficient than mature grass. Low soil Mg of heavy application of K rich fertilizers in pasture may lead to Mg availability to grass and subsequently to the animal lead to grass tetany. Other factors like excessive production of ammonia in rumen prevents absorption of Mg, reduction of dry feed intake etc may lead to grass tetany among the livestock.

Treatment

1. Administration of Mg salt like MgSO4 (10-20%) @ 200-300 ml (s/c route).
2. Mifex @ 1 bottle (500 ml through i/v route and 500 ml through route).
3. Mg gluconate 15% solution @ 200-300 ml s/c route.

10.4.6 Mineral and trace element deficiency

Problems of mineral or trace element deficiency or imbalance are not specifically reported in the literature from yak-producing countries. Copper supplementation of the yak diet and occasional copper injection has brought improvement in the health, vigour and performance of the yak. This suggests at least the possibility that yak may have an inadequate copper uptake due to an inherently low capacity of yak to absorb dietary copper - because a genetic component to the uptake of copper is well documented in other species. Claus and Dierenfeld (1999) have reviewed and discussed the topic and provided more evidence of copper deficiency in captive yak.

Copper deficiency can result in poor growth and poor fertility, among other symptoms - but poor growth and poor fertility, by themselves, do not necessarily indicate copper or any other mineral or trace element deficiency, as overall poor nutrition may be the cause of the problem. In actual mineral and trace element deficiencies, appropriate supplementation will generally improve the conditions caused.

References

Biswas, D., Barari, S.K. & Pal, R.N. (1994). Ticks and lice infestations in yak. Proceedings of the first International Congress on Yak. *Journal of Gansu agricultural University* (Special issue, June, 1994), pp. 322-324.

Claus, M. & Dierenfeld, E.S. (1999). Susceptibility of yak (*Bos grunniens*) to copper deficiency. *The Veterinary Record,* 145, 436-437

Joshi, D.D. (1982). *Yak and chauri Husbandry in Nepal.* H.M. Government Press, Singha, Nepal.

Joshi, D.D. *et al.* (1997). Epidemiological aspects of yak diseases in Nepal. *Proceedings of the second international congress on yak, in Xining, China, 1-6 September 1997.*

Lensch, J (1996). Krankheiten: In *Der Yak (Bos grunniens) in Zentralasien* (eds. Jurgen Lensch, Peter Schley and Rong-Chang Zhang). Duncker & Humblot. Berlin 1996, pp 237-246.

Liu, W.D. (1994). Observations on growth-decline rule of roundworm and its larva in yak's stomach and intestine. Proceedings of the first international congress on yak. *Journal of Gansu Agricultural University.* (Special issue, June 1994), pp. 339-342.

Pal, R.N. (1993). Domestic yak *(Poephagus grunniens* L.): A research review. *Indian Journal of Animal Sciences,* 63, 743-753.

Rahman, H, Bhattacharya, M, Rajkhowa, J, Soud, N, Nandankar,U, Mukherjee, S. (2007a). Seroprevalence of brucellosis in yaks (*Poephagus grunniens*) in India. Ind. J. Anim. Sci., 77: 796-798.

Rahman, H, Bhattacharya, M, Rajkhowa, J, Soud, N, Nandankar,U, Mukherjee, S. (2007b). Seroprevalence of infectious rhinotrachitis in yaks (*Poephagus grunniens*) in India. Ind. J. Anim. Sci., 77: 793-795.

Rahman,H., Chatlod, L.R., Pal, P. and Rahman, H. (2009). Diseases of yak (Poephagus grunniens)- An overview. Proc. Of International conference on yak husbandry- challenges and strategies. NRC on yak (ICAR), Dirang, Arunachal Pradesh. India.

Wangdi, P. (1996). Survey of gid eradication program: incidence of coenurosis in yak population at Lingshe dungkahg. *Yak Newsletter* (Volume no. 2, November, 1996), pp. 12-24.

Yu J.F. *et al.*, (1989). Investigation on bovine *babesiasis* of yak. *Journal of China Yak*, 1, 40-42.

❑❑❑

Chapter 11

Future Research and Conclusion

Yak *(Poephagus grunniens)*, a close relative of cattle, is one of the world's most remarkable domestic ruminant as it thrives in conditions of extreme harshness and unfriendly weather conditions while providing a livelihood security for millions of people in high altitudes. Long wooly hair makes them very attractive and it is necessary for thriving in their natural habitat at altitudes of 3000-5000 m or more as in Tibetan plateau and part of Arunachal Pradesh, Sikkim and Ladakh region of Jammu & Kashmir, Lahul and Spiti of Himachal Pradesh. The distinctive grunt produced by these animals during mating season gives them the systematic name of *Poephagus grunniens*. Yak is a very sturdy animal and may negotiate and graze in areas normally inaccessible to hardiest cattle breed. Role of yak in higher elevations as pack animal, source of milk, meat and their byproducts and rearing requires almost nothing except winter months feeding. This also carries a symbol of prosperity of Tibetan Buddhism and signifies religious and cultural sentiment.

Yak population in India are scattered and there is urgent need to type characterization of the species inhabiting different places and to ascertain the genetic diversity among them. Yak products like milk by products, meat by products, horn and hooves, skin and hide and most importantly hair must be commercialized in the region. Yak are facing danger as often the younger population is showing interest for other avenues like small business or tourist guide that are readily available and giving money in a small period of time. This indicates the rearing of yak must be make more profitable and market oriented by the scientists working in the field. At the same time shrinkage of habitat due to deforestation, industrialization, increased human population, global warming may be other attributes for decline yak population globally.

The research is thus needed to conserve the yak and improvement of economic trait of the animal and survival of the species and livelihood security of people related to it. Genetic improvement may be done through selection of superior yak bull. Though under nomadic system of yak rearing it is very difficult, elite animals may be selected by judging the individual performance, pedigree and type conformity. Once elite herd of yak is established, then it will be easier to improve genetic potentiality of the yak. At the same time, interspecies hybridization is long been practiced by the local people and can be continued for the improvement in milk production to retains its economic importance. One drawback of the hybridization is that the male hybrids are always sterile and poor adaptability in higher altitudes, however, they have higher draught power. Females are superior milk producer. Hybridization of yak with local cattle is one of the most important factor for declining pure yak population across the world.

Yak milk has known to have therapeutic and medicinal value due to physiologically active component as maintained on grasses, natural fodders and other fauna under organic system by default mostly in higher elevations. Therapeutic and medicinal quality of milk, meat and other byproducts needs to be investigated scientifically and at the same time traditional old age practice of processing the products into byproducts needs to be investigated for improvement. Small yak milk processing unit for development of entrepreneurship, dissemination of technologies for production of value added milk products from yak like *dahi, paneer, khoa,* flavoured milk and *lassi,* whey beverages and milk sweets which can increase the income by many folds. Government support is very much essential to investigate the matter and develop proper marketing facilities of the yak milk and milk products.

Though large number of molecular markers associated with economically important traits has been identified in cattle, sheep, goat and pigs, such markers are yet to be identified in yak. Under these circumstances short term molecular markers could be used for parentage identification and genetic diversity studies.

At the same time, conservation is needed keeping in mind its uniqueness, multifarious usefulness and above all essentiality of highlanders under the prevailing cultural and socio-economic- religious conditions. Research is needed to study ecological balance and natural selection of breeding, suitable breeding policies for economic upliftment of the herdsmen. Multi-purpose breeding objectives must be kept in mind and economic efficiency of yak has to be measured on the basis of overall overall lifetime profitability. It is desirable to carry out well designed hybridization programme outside the conservation zone to improve performance of yak hybrids and overall income of yak farmers. Feed scarcity is another most serious problem in the high altitude. Especially during severe winter feed availability nearly nil. Still they are surviving and performing to the nutritional harsh condition. Provision of feeds to that scarcity period is the challenging task to the farmer as well as researchers. Nutritional interventions are also needed to improve the body condition, performance and functional food preparation at grassroot level. Rumen manipulation is needed to study the microbial diversity, nature and prevalence as well as role of feed additives for the improvement of the production performance in yak.

As yak are raised under transhumance system of animal rearing, managemental intervention to improve the performance of the animals is not a easy task. However, reproduction management during summer and feeding management especially winter months play important role for the overall performance of the domesticated yak. Yak does not need elaborate shelter. They can thrive well in the harsh climatic conditions. Prevalence of diseases is limited due to their natural habitat. However, deficiency diseases are not uncommon.

In the last few decades, various research programme has been initiated towards yak. Application of advanced biotechnological tools may help to solve basic problems related to the production and reproduction. Although yaks are less susceptible to the diseases, but diseases can be prevented with the adoption of preventive measures time to time.

Keeping the view of changes in environmental indices especially global warming, as these are highest dwelling animals must have some effect on survival as well as on biological parameters. Need of the hour is to study its effect, so that effect on other animals and mankind may be predicted to prevent such situation. Effect on global warming on natural pastures and meadows are also be studied for improvement and prevention. Without yak human civilization at this high altitude may be questionable in future.

❑❑❑

About the Authors

Dr. Goutam Mondal is working as Scientist (Senior Scale) at Mountain Research Centre for Sheep & Goat, S K University of Agricultural Sciences & Technology- Kashmir, Shuhama, Srinagar. He has worked in Ladakh for more than 6 years. He graduated from West Bengal University of Animal Fishery Sciences, Kolkata and Masters and Ph.D. from National Dairy Research Institute, Karnal, Haryana. The author is engaged in teaching, research and extension work in undergraduate student and field level. He has published more than 50 articles in national and international journal of repute. He has published one book and one book chapter. Current area of research is ruminant nutrition with special reference to feed fortification for better utilization in animal system.

Dr. Biswajit Roy is presently working as Associate Professor in the Department of Livestock Production and Management, College of Veterinary Science and Animal Husbandry, Madhya Pradesh Pashu Chikitsa Vigyan Vishwa Vidyalaya (MPPCVV), Jabalpur, Madhya Pradesh. He obtained B.V.Sc. & A.H. from West Bengal University of Animal Fishery Sciences, Kolkata and master and Ph.D. from National Dairy Research Institute, Karnal, Haryana. He obtained MBA (HRM) degree from IGNOU, New Delhi. He is actively engaged in research and teaching of undergraduate, masters and doctoral students. So far he has published more than 50 research paper, reviews and popular article in the national and international journals.

Dr. Biswajit Brahma is working as Jr. Scientist (Livestock Production and Management) in Krishi Vigyan Kendra, Bhadarwah, S K University of Agricultural Sciences and Technology -Jammu for last several years. He obtained B.V.Sc & AH from West Bengal University of Animal And Fishery Sciences, Kolkota and M.V.Sc from National Dairy Research Institute, Karnal, Haryana. He has been actively engaged in research and extension work on livestock management in hilly areas. His present research area includes molecular characterization of Yak-Cattle hybrids and genetic diversity of innate immunity in Indian Cattle & Buffalo.

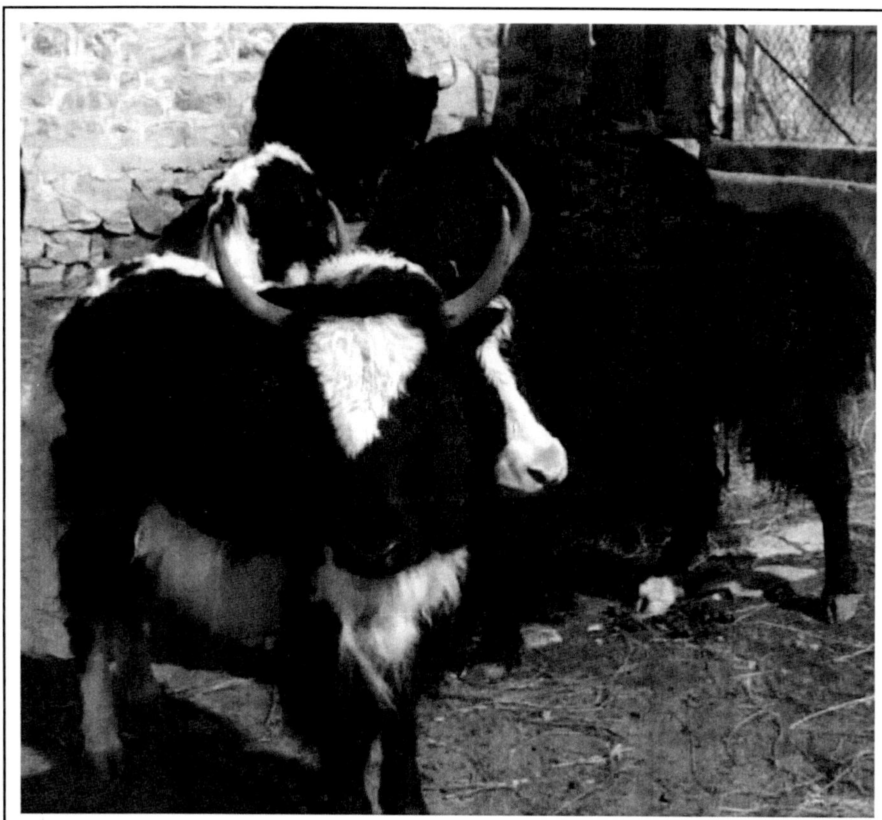

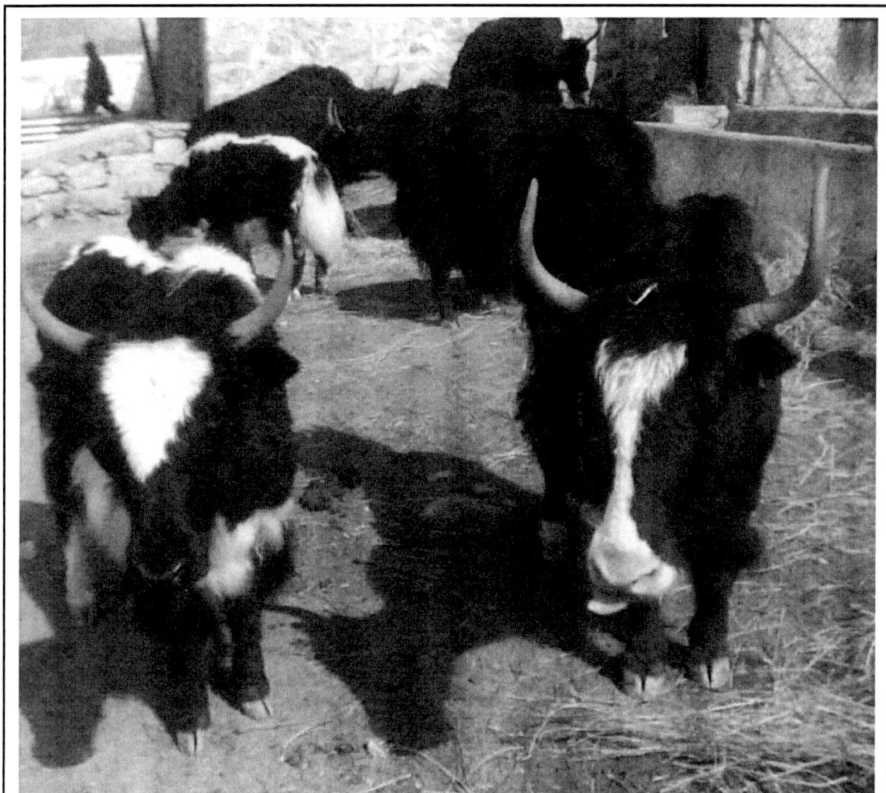

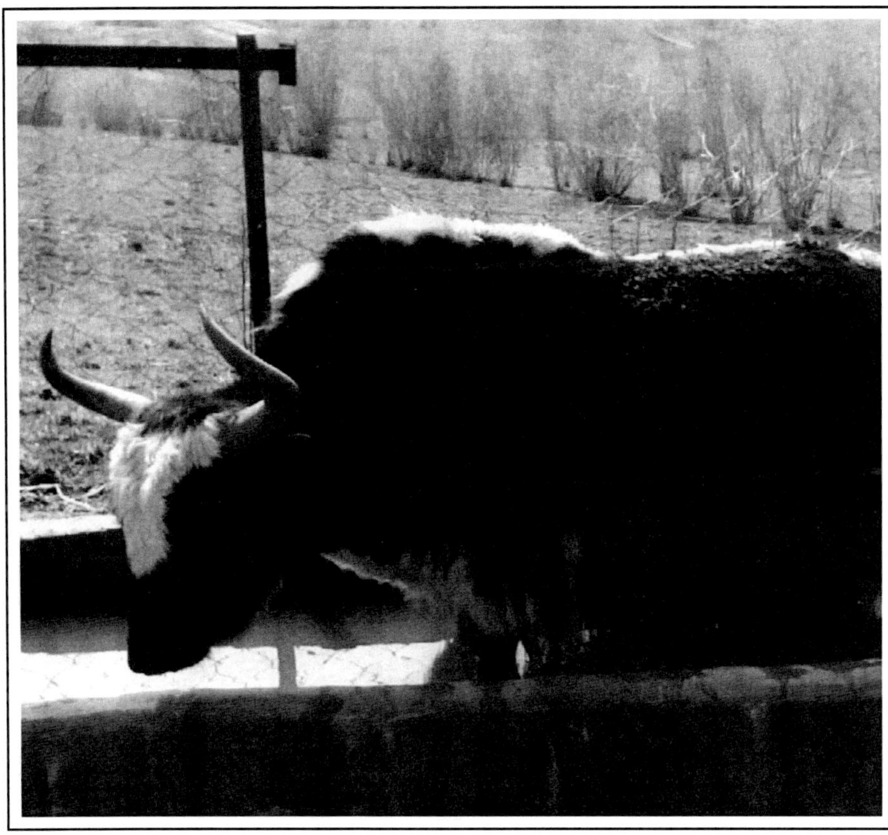

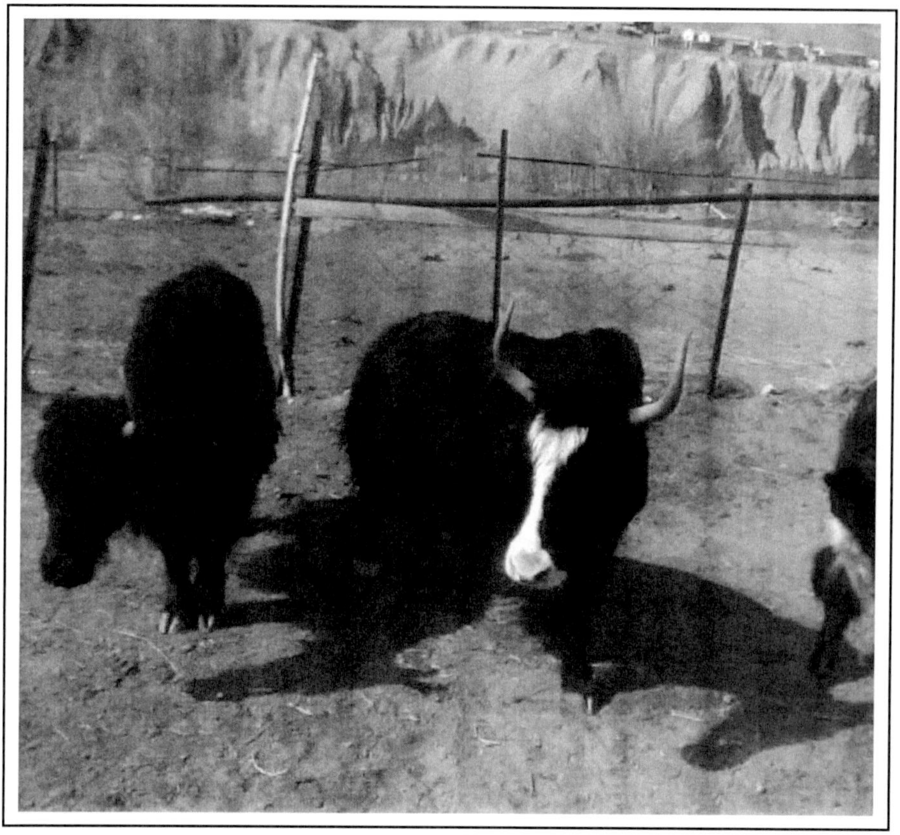

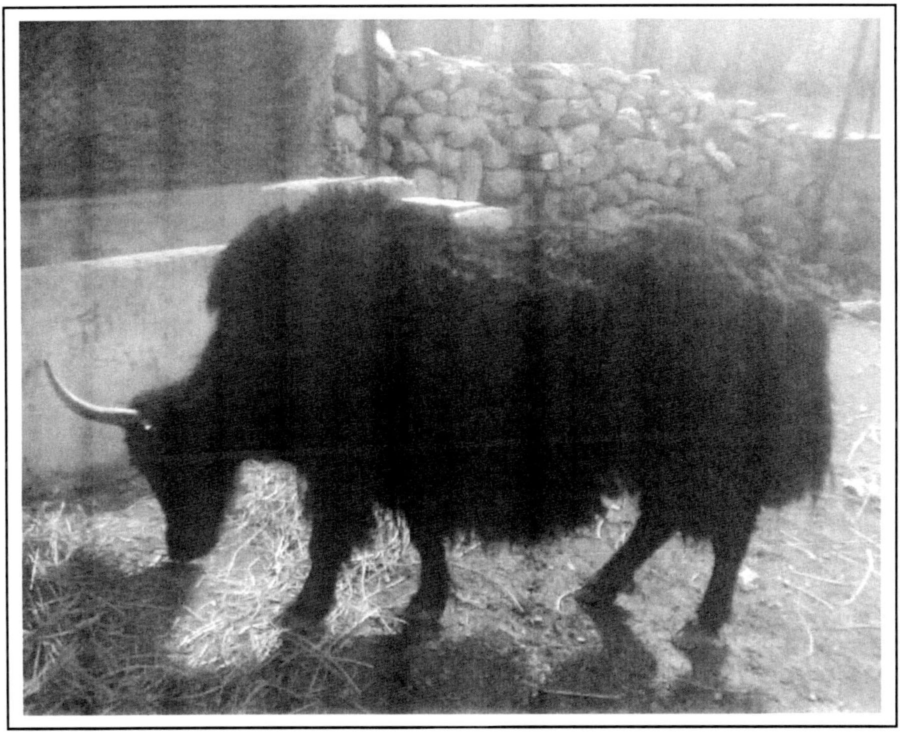

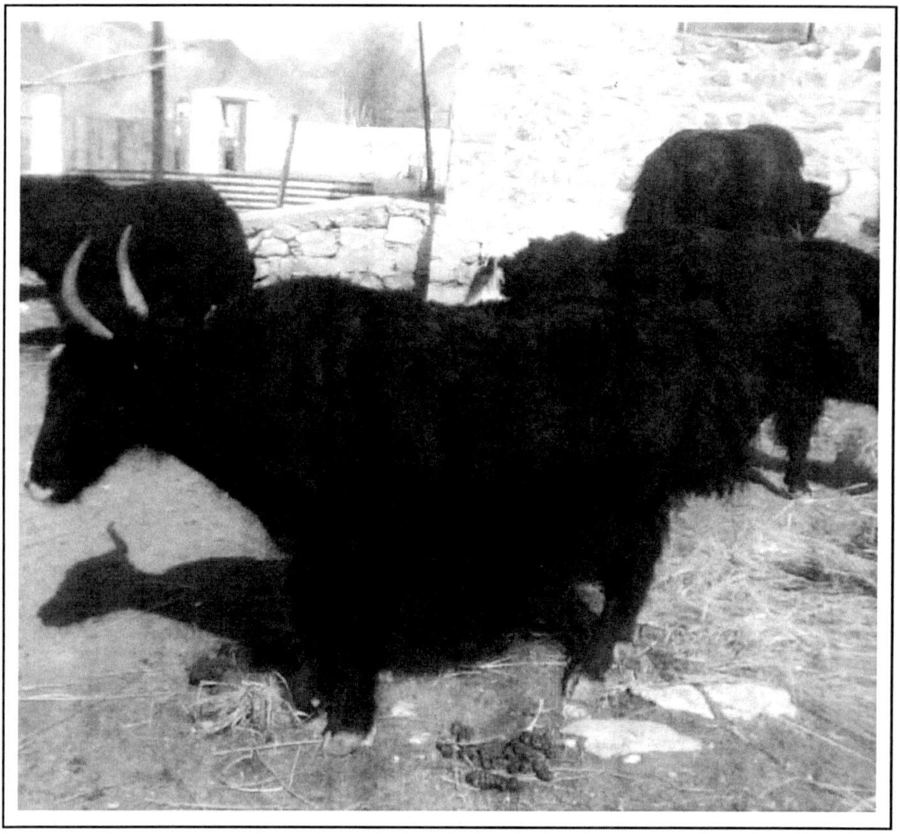

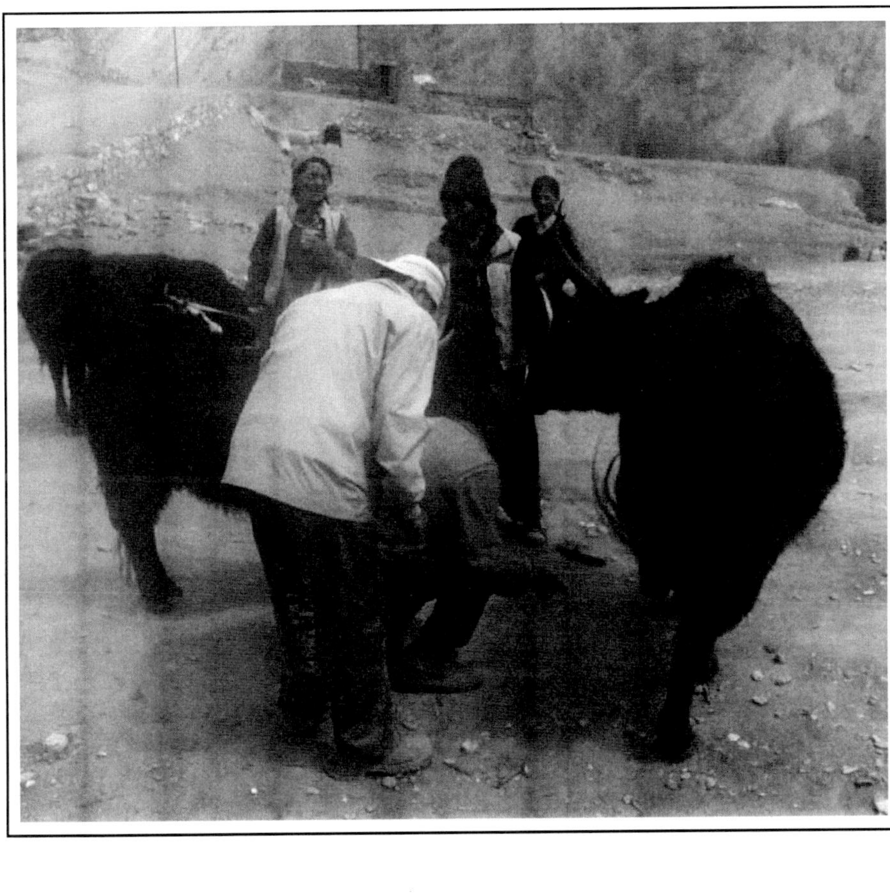

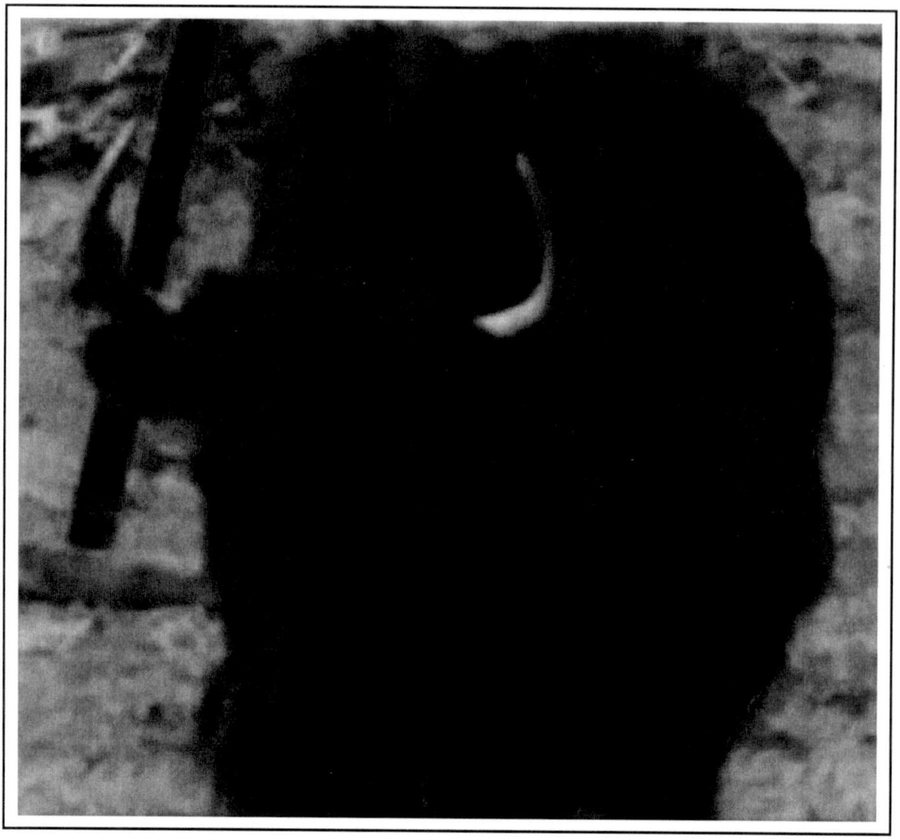

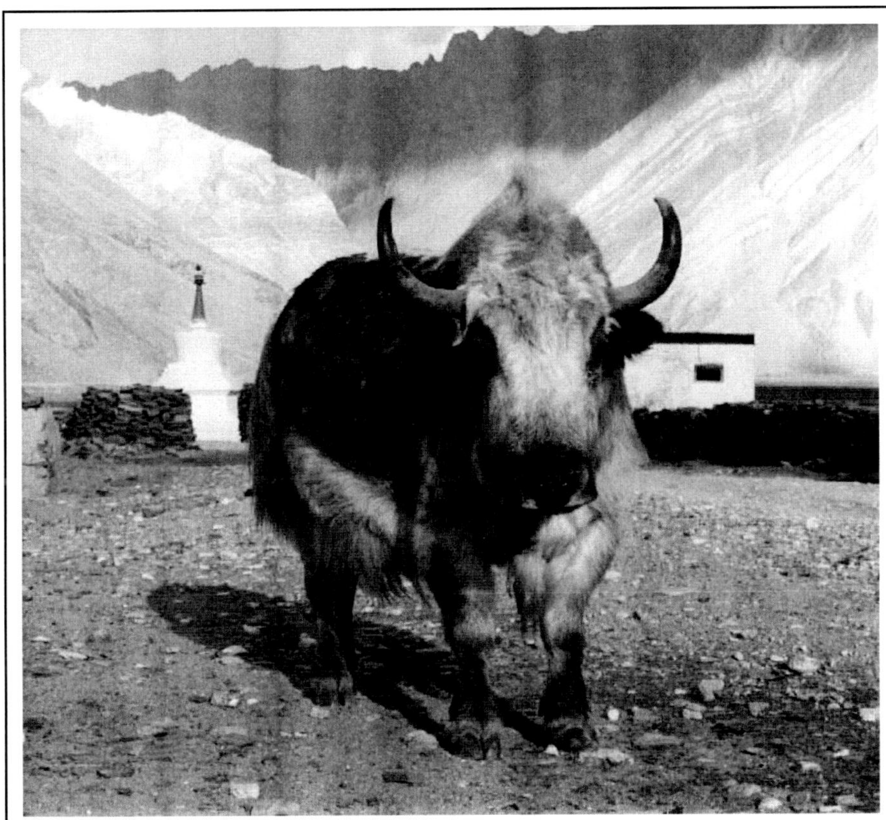

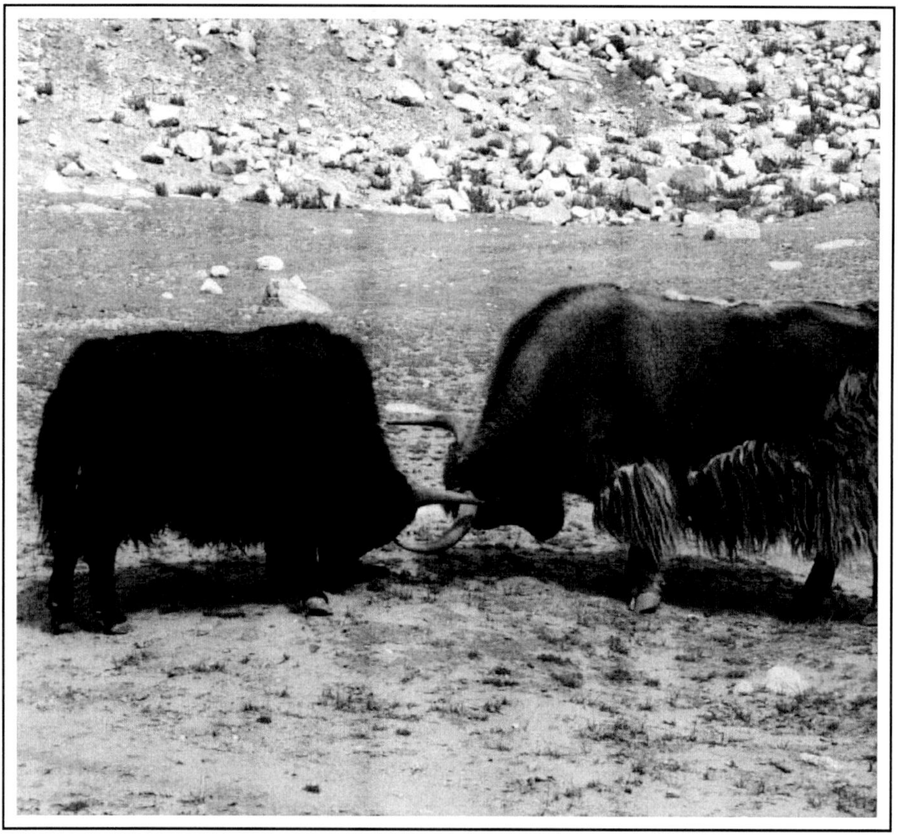